GOD'S HANDS NOT MINE

Norma Garrett

NORMA GARRETT
with
DEBBIE RONK

ISBN 978-1-63525-188-3 (Paperback)
ISBN 978-1-63525-187-6 (Digital)

Copyright © 2016 by Norma Garrett and Debbie Ronk
All rights reserved. No part of this publication may be reproduced, distributed, or transmitted in any form or by any means, including photocopying, recording, or other electronic or mechanical methods without the prior written permission of the publisher. For permission requests, solicit the publisher via the address below.

Christian Faith Publishing, Inc.
296 Chestnut Street
Meadville, PA 16335
www.christianfaithpublishing.com

Printed in the United States of America

During the final days of this writing process,
my sweet mama was delivered into the arms of Jesus,
and reunited with my precious daddy…

I dedicate this book to the honor and memory of my parents,
for they clearly exemplified a life of
Godly love and sacrifice.

Contents

Preface 7
Chapter 1 In God's Hands 9
Chapter 2 Welcome to My World 12
Chapter 3 Playing, My Way 15
Chapter 4 School Days 19
Chapter 5 Stepping toward Normalcy 22
Chapter 6 Valley of Miracles 25
Chapter 7 Teamwork Brings Honors 29
Chapter 8 Seeking New Heights 32
Chapter 9 Persistence Paves the Way 35
Chapter 10 Feet at Work 39
Chapter 11 Prisoners Give Freedom 44
Chapter 12 My Father's Hands 58
Chapter 13 Milkshake Made in Heaven 62
Chapter 14 Together in Love 66
Chapter 15 Married with Children 69

Chapter 16	Time on the Lake	72
Chapter 17	Unexpected Changes	74
Chapter 18	Major Adjustments	77
Chapter 19	Searching for Purpose	81
Chapter 20	Trying Times	84
Chapter 21	Hope	86
Chapter 22	Seniors on the Go	88
Chapter 23	Reversal of Roles	90
Chapter 24	God's Hands, Not Mine	93

PREFACE

The telling of my life story has been a work in progress for more than twenty-four years. It was my Dad who initially planted the idea. There have been six different assistants throughout this process, with long lapses of time between each of them. In 2012, God led me to Debbie, who had been called to serve Him through her writing. Feeling God's presence, Debbie and I began working together knowing that God does not call the qualified to do His work, but qualifies those He calls. This book is a result of trusting and seeking the Lord's guidance every step of the way. No doubt, God's timing has been hugely instrumental in bringing about the final outcome. To God be the glory and praise!

I would like to thank all of those who have prayed for Debbie and me. God has used you greatly to support and cheer us on. I also thank all those who have loved and accepted me throughout my not-so-normal life. Although each name cannot be mentioned here, you know who you are and the part you had in helping me accomplish my dreams.

My special husband, Kenneth, has been the greatest supporter of all. He has worked behind the scenes as a constant voice of encouragement. Kenneth has always loved and cared for me in ways that most men would never consider; and I am so thankful for his presence in my life.

Most of all, I thank God for His ever present faithfulness. My thoughts and feelings are best expressed through one of my favorite songs, "My Tribute."

My Tribute

How can I say thanks for the things You have done for me?
Things so undeserved, yet You gave to prove Your love for me.
The voices of a million angels could not express my gratitude.
All that I am and ever hope to be, I owe it all to Thee.
To God be the glory, to God be the glory,
To God be the glory for the things He has done.
With His blood He has saved me.
With His power He has raised me.
To God be the glory for the things He has done.
Just let me live my life—let it be pleasing, Lord, to Thee.
And if I gain any praise, let it go to Calvary.
With His blood He has saved me.
With His power He has raised me.
To God be the glory for the things He has done.

CHAPTER 1

In God's Hands

For you created my inmost being; you knit me together in my mother's womb.
Psalm 139:13

After six years of marriage, my parents were anxiously awaiting the arrival of their first child. On Christmas Eve 1944, I "chimed" into this world as carols were echoing through the hallways of the Roanoke Memorial Hospital in Virginia. It was almost noon on Sunday. There had been no reason to expect anything out of the ordinary concerning my arrival. My mother was healthy throughout her pregnancy and carried me full term. She and Dad were eagerly awaiting the moment to hold their baby in their arms.

Moments after the delivery, while Mom was under sedation, the doctor approached my dad in the waiting room. He explained to him that his five pound fourteen ounce newborn baby girl had come into the world with multiple birth defects. I was born with no arms, and my right leg was shorter and underdeveloped. My right foot, with only four toes, was bent to the side so far that my pinky nearly touched my leg. Neither of my hips had fully developed ball joints, and my back was not properly aligned. Even the knee joint of my left leg was not fully developed. In addition, I had a partial cleft palate. The doctor felt that I would be pretty helpless and a lifetime burden to everyone. Offering little encouragement or hope for my future, he suggested that my parents consider placing me in an institution.

With so much to process, Dad immediately left the hospital and went to my great-aunt and uncle's house. Uncle Gurney was the pastor of the Presbyterian Church where my parents were faithful members. Dad, Uncle Gurney, and Aunt Lece discussed the situation at hand. Aunt Lece expressed with certainty that God knew what he was doing when He placed me in this particular family. So, together they prayed at length for God's help and placed me in His hands. Upon returning to the hospital, the doctor asked my father what he planned to do. Dad responded, "Well, the first thing I am going to do is get a new doctor."

There was no known medical or scientific explanation for my birth defects. The doctor and my dad were afraid the unexpected news might be detrimental to my mother's healing process, so they chose to wait until she was feeling physically and emotionally stronger to share the information.

As my mother gradually regained her strength, she began to suspect that something was wrong. Whenever she asked to see her baby she was given numerous reasons why they couldn't bring me to her room. It was not until I was four days old that she was told of my condition and allowed to hold me. Her mind was filled with thoughts, concerns, and questions; but her heart was only filled with love for her baby girl. Although Dad and the doctor had been trying to protect her, they had clearly underestimated her ability to handle the circumstances. Not one tear was shed nor did she respond in any negative way. She was simply thankful to be given such a blessing, and eager to become acquainted with her newborn child.

Knowing I would arrive around the Christmas holiday, my parents had planned to name me Noel. However, unable to find a middle name that they really liked to go along with Noel, they decided to name me Norma Ellen instead.

Becoming new parents always brings its own set of challenges, but for my parents, the challenges were somewhat different. Their daughter had special needs and would require more than the usual attention, care, and love. They would seek the help they needed, one day at a time. My mom and dad took me into their arms and into their hearts with the assurance that God would help them.

Chapter 2

Welcome to My World

*I praise you because I am fearfully and
wonderfully made.
Psalm 139:14a*

Upon returning home from the hospital, Mom was fortunate to receive help from a lady in our church, Mrs. Jacobs, who stayed with us for several weeks. As a new mother, there were many duties and responsibilities to accomplish each day. Not to mention that cloth diapers needed to be laundered and hung on a line along with other clothing; dryers were a luxury at that time. Mom naturally accepted the role of primary caregiver and homemaker while Dad provided financially through his job with the railroad. His position often required double-shift hours and daytime sleeping.

Mrs. Jacobs also sewed a few baby outfits for me, including some feed-sack dresses. Yes, clothes were actually made from cotton chickenfeed sacks. All the dresses that I wore had sleeves in them. Oftentimes, they were puffed short sleeves. It probably didn't occur to Mom to have the sleeves altered, or maybe she liked the way the sleeves broadened my narrow shoulders. In all my baby pictures I look like most babies, smiling and wearing a frilly dress, and a hair bow that Mom always placed on top of my head. I honestly don't know how she managed to keep the bow in my baby fine hair.

WELCOME TO MY WORLD

I did exactly what all babies do, crying when I was wet or hungry. Otherwise, I was a happy baby, smiled a lot, and cooed my way into everyone's hearts. Although there were physical differences in my appearance, I was otherwise a perfectly healthy child. Mom and Dad naturally began taking me to church when I was three to four weeks old. Much like home, the people at Belmont Presbyterian were very loving and supportive.

During the infant stage of my life, Mom instinctively initiated her own form of physical therapy on my right foot by gradually manipulating its angle to a more natural position. This act of love has enabled me to use that foot in daily living activities much more than would ever have been possible.

When I was six months old, I started grasping playthings with my left foot. I gripped other's fingers and would grab objects with my foot as naturally as any child does with his or her hands. I was simply using what I had. I should mention that I had also been blessed with an incredible amount of energy and curiosity.

Before I learned to "crawl," I perfected rolling. I could roll quite rapidly in any direction I wanted to go. This skill really tickled my parents, providing them with more than your usual baby entertainment. Later on, I scooted to get from place to place, by sitting on my bottom and shifting from side to side while pulling myself forward with my legs.

During my toddler stage, getting from one place to another was never a problem. Unfortunately, ready-made wheelchairs to fit my unique physique were not available; Dad's ingenuity, skills, and determination, however, always provided a creative solution. He happily accepted the challenge to invent some means of mobility to fit my various stages of development and more. First, there was the rectangular padded seat with four swivel wheels on which I scooted myself around. I soon graduated to three and four wheel strollers that I propelled quite well with my left foot. When not using "Dad's wheels," I would "waddle" short distances to get around indoors. Later in preschool years, Dad built my first wheelchair from a child's rocking chair. He removed the rockers and placed the chair on a flat platform with two swivel wheels in the front and two stable wheels in the back.

My feet became my hands and were rarely covered with socks or shoes. With practice and determination I developed strength, dexterity, and flexibility in my toes and feet. By the age of two, I was learning to feed myself. I would prop my left leg on a higher surface, hold a spoon between my toes, then bend down towards the spoon to eat. When performing this feat my left knee would automatically bend backwards making this easier to accomplish. There were many messes for Mom to clean up, but maybe her patience was strengthened by her relief that I was discovering my own ways to be independent. I simply did what was natural for me in order to accomplish what I saw everyone else doing.

I could feed myself, but needed Mom's help with most of my personal care and hygiene. Although I was able to comb my hair and brush my teeth using the same method I used for eating, she bathed and dressed me, and assisted me in the bathroom. Due to my small size, Mom was able to carry me around on her hip more easily while accomplishing these tasks.

Mom also took care of altering my clothes—shortening pant legs and sleeves, while hemming skirts and dresses—as needed to fit my frame. She gave of herself willingly and often sacrificially. In her words, she was simply doing whatever was necessary to get the job done. If Mom had any emotional adjustments that come with having a child with special needs, it certainly didn't show. I never felt any reluctance or resentment from her. There were times when Mom felt the curious stares of strangers, but she quickly learned to overlook them and move on. She was a strong woman who was not easily discouraged.

CHAPTER 3

Playing, My Way

*Honor your father and mother…that it may
go well with you and that you may
enjoy long life on the earth.
Ephesians 6:2–3*

When I was sixteen months old, my mother gave birth to a perfectly normal healthy baby boy. Barry had blue eyes and fuzzy blonde hair. In fact, his hair was so blonde and fine that he appeared bald for several months. With a new addition to the family, we all had to make adjustments. I was no longer the only child getting Mom and Dad's sole attention. On one occasion, when my aunt Mae was babysitting the two of us, Barry began to cry. Before Aunt Mae could get to him, I had quickly rolled across the floor to console Barry by rocking his cradle gently with my foot. I was only two at that time, but clearly my actions showed my acceptance and love for my baby brother.

In general, Barry's and my relationship was typical of brothers and sisters. Although I had additional needs, Mom and Dad found a healthy balance while giving attention to both of us. Neither Barry nor I suffered from overprotection or lack of love or discipline.

Because Dad worked long hours on the railroad, Mom was responsible for most of the discipline in our home. She taught us right from wrong and applied the appropriate response to encourage the desired behavior. Mom knew how to use a switch when it was necessary, but more often she was known for "pinching" when she needed to let us know she meant business. Although I was physically handicapped, I was treated no differently when it came to disciplinary action. Mom recognized the importance of appropriate punishment, and demonstrated her love by setting firm boundaries. Her keen nurturing instincts combined with Dad's "you can do it" encouragement provided the balanced environment needed particularly for my early physical and mental development.

I often pulled rank on Barry, asserting my "older sister" status. Sometimes I was even caught intimidating and bullying him. When I was five or six years old, I backed him into a small space between the stove and refrigerator daring him to move. When he tried to escape, I smacked at him with my left foot in an attempt to show him who was boss. When Barry cried out in protest, we both found out who was really in charge; Mom, of course.

When my brother and all the neighborhood children were playing outside, I was right out there with them. We played hopscotch, Mother May I, kickball, and many other typical children's games. When there was a need to improvise, my playmates accepted my way of adapting without protest or hesitation.

It never occurred to me that there might be some things I couldn't do. I just took for granted that I could do anything I set my mind to, and I pretty much did. For instance, I played hopscotch while sitting in my wheelchair by first tossing the rock into the appropriate square with my foot. Then, getting a rolling start, I passed over the hopscotch squares on the sidewalk touching each square quickly with only my left foot. If I missed a square or touched a line, I was out just like anyone else. Another activity I enjoyed was roller skating. While in my chair, I would attach a roller skate to my left shoe and roll down the hill beside our house. I was able to guide my wheelchair by pointing the skate in the direction I wanted to go. I got quite adept at slowing down my momentum by turning my skate from left to right. I was able to stop myself from going into the street by rolling off into the grass. It didn't matter to me that I could only skate downhill or that I was sitting in my chair while doing it. I was roller skating with the rest of the kids and that was all that mattered.

When I was not outside playing, my best friends Carolyn and Judi would often visit. We usually played cards, played board games, colored pictures, or cut out paper dolls. No one ever seemed surprised that I could use scissors with my toes. One of our favorite things was pretending to be "mommies" to our baby dolls, often making playhouses and restaurants out of large appliance boxes.

In the winter months, I thoroughly enjoyed playing in the snow and eating homemade snow cream. I remember one particular winter when it snowed on the same day several weeks in a row. Forty inches had accumulated and I couldn't wait to go outside. Mom bundled me up for my snowy day adventure. When more than sufficiently dressed in multiple layers of clothing, Dad took me out the front door and literally "flung" me into the air. I was laughing excitedly as I landed on my back, sinking into the deep snow. I then made a snow angel, only without wings.

Dad made a side-board frame to fit our sled to prevent me from falling off while riding down bumpy snow-packed hills. I don't suppose sledding was quite as much fun for my brother since he was often the one to get me back to the top for another ride. Barry seldom complained, although I'm sure there were plenty of times he would rather have been with his friends instead of helping me.

During the summer months, our family often spent time at a cabin on the Roanoke River. We mostly played outdoor games like horseshoes and crochet, but playing in the cold river was probably one of our favorite activities. Dad figured out a way to make me safely independent in the water, so that I could participate in the fun. He fastened twine around an inner tube and made webbing across the opening to provide a seat for me. When he sat me in it, I floated all by myself. I could go anywhere I wanted in the water by paddling with my feet, and leaning in one direction or the other. However, during one of our river adventures, I must have been bobbing up and down a little too energetically, and tipped over my floating vessel. I found myself upside down with my head and body under water, and my legs kicking frantically in the air. As I held my breath, I could see the legs of everyone standing around me. I hoped someone would quickly notice my predicament and rescue me. Thankfully, not long into the kicking, I felt my dad's hands turning me right side up. Despite this scary experience, my enthusiasm for playing in the water was not "dampened".

CHAPTER 4

School Days

With God all things are possible.
Matthew 19:26b

At the age of six, my friends and I were very excited to start school. Since kindergarten was not required at that time, we would be entering the first grade. My enthusiasm quickly diminished when I was told I would not be able to attend public school. This was such a shock and disappointment since I had never before felt excluded from anything. It was the first time in my life that I truly felt *different*.

Developmentally, I was just like any other child my age. However, because of my physical limitations, I received instruction for several hours each weekday in my home. My bedroom became my classroom when Dad hung a chalkboard on the wall, and my first grade teacher was quite surprised at what I already knew. Despite this observation, she wrote on my report card that I would always be a homebound student.

My second and third grade teacher, Mrs. Meador, had a different outlook concerning my education. She often took me to the corner store as part of my math instruction. I think her real goal was to get me out in public to interact with other people. We would buy candy, but I was expected to do all the talking and purchasing. She taught me a lot more than reading, writing, and arithmetic. Through her instruction, I was also developing self-confidence and social skills.

By the end of my third year, Mrs. Meador had recognized my potential and felt confident that I could be successfully mainstreamed into the public school system. She talked with my parents about a school across town that provided teacher's aides and accessibility for handicapped students. My mom had concerns about the assistance I would need for personal care, but at the same time she recognized the opportunity for interacting with other children. Therefore, with Dad's positive encouragement, she agreed to let me go to "real" school.

Transportation was provided for handicapped students, and as I boarded the bus heading for West End Elementary School, I experienced both the excitement and fears usually associated with going to school. I did need some personal assistance, but otherwise was placed in a regular classroom. My special desk without legs was always placed on the floor of the front row to give me an unobstructed view of the teacher and the chalkboard.

I loved school; loved being with other kids and made friends easily. At first, other children stared at me. Some asked, "What happened to your arms?" I would laugh and say, "Nothing! I never had any." After satisfying their curiosity, we would often get acquainted and become friends.

It was during my first year in public school that I met Joanna. She was also dependent on a wheelchair, but her circumstances were very different. Joanna had been paralyzed from the waist down due to a horse riding accident. We shared the same birthday, but she was one year younger. Joanna and I soon discovered we had many of the same interests and became close friends, spending countless hours giggling and talking at school and on the phone. When I visited her home, I was surprised to see her large collection of horse statues. Joanna still loved horses despite her debilitating accident.

Spending time with Joanna and her mom during the Christmas season was especially enjoyable. Decorating their Christmas tree and helping her mom with baking were among my favorite activities. Making fudge topped the list. My job was stirring the chocolate mixture which was done by holding a spoon in one foot while steadying the bowl with the other. Once the fudge was poured into a pan, Joanna and I were allowed to lick the spoons. That was our favorite part. Being handicapped doesn't mean that you can't have fun, and Joanna and I had our share of it. When others seemed uncomfortable around us, we simply smiled at them, made eye contact, and initiated a conversation. We liked to laugh and make others laugh, too.

In addition to classroom instruction, the special education students at West End were offered swimming lessons at the YWCA. I quickly jumped at this opportunity. The school provided transportation to the Y, and once we arrived each student was assigned a personal assistant in the pool. After overcoming any fear of the water, we were taught how to float. My natural buoyancy made this easy for me. After accomplishing this, we were taught other swimming techniques. By kicking my feet I could swim in any direction I wanted to go while at the same time compensating for the different lengths of my legs. By rotating my left leg in a circular motion, I could roll myself over to swim on my back or face down. Swimming was a lot of fun and another way that I could be like everyone else.

After completing six years at West End, I looked forward to my years at Jackson Junior High School. However, because there were no elevators, those that could not climb stairs were unable to attend. Instead, a "homebound" teacher was assigned to teach us at West End. This was another huge disappointment, but at least I was still "going to school."

CHAPTER 5

Stepping toward Normalcy

*Man looks at the outward appearance,
but the Lord looks at the heart.
1 Samuel 16:7b*

My parents began taking me to regularly scheduled appointments at a local clinic to meet with orthopedic specialists when I was very young. Dr. Bray was my favorite doctor—a warm and caring man who always showed a personal interest in me. When I was approximately eight years old, Dr. Bray and his team members suggested that fitting me with artificial arms might make me *appear* more normal. They recommended that I go to Kessler Institute, a well-established rehabilitation center, located in West Orange, New Jersey. The procedure would require several weeks all together. It was a difficult decision to make due to my age and the separation from home and family. However, because Mom, Dad, and I felt it was important to explore all options available, we proceeded with the necessary arrangements.

The time came for my parents and me to make the long trip to New Jersey. Being only nine years old at the time, it seemed to take forever. We stayed in a motel that evening in West Orange, and arrived at the rehab center the following morning. During our initial meeting with the doctors at Kessler, they explained the operational procedure for fitting me with arms. In order to use the prosthetic arms it was necessary to surgically insert a short rod through a hole under each collarbone. Functionally, from my perspective, as well as my parents, there seemed to be no benefit to attaching artificial arms other than making me *look* more like everyone else. The changes would not enable me to do anything that I wasn't already doing. When we rejected this idea, the Kessler staff suggested that a prosthetic leg be made that would enable me to walk. We liked this idea and gave the doctors permission to move forward in the planning process.

After my parents met the staff, toured the residence, and settled me into my new "home away from home," they said their good-byes and headed back to Roanoke. They appeared to be strong and reassuring as they prepared to leave; however, they were so upset with leaving me, that tears were shed and not a word was spoken for at least the first hour during their trip back home.

My stay at Kessler Institute took place during the summer. Being on my own and so far from home and family for the first time in my life was kind of scary. However, there was plenty to do, which made the time go by quickly. In addition to my scheduled therapies, there were many fun recreational activities in which to participate. Shuffleboard was among my favorite.

Initially a stiltlike brace was made to fit my right leg, so that both my legs would be the same length. With daily physical, occupational, and recreational therapy, I gained the strength needed for walking with this apparatus. It required a lot of practice, effort, and patience to accomplish this goal.

In the meantime, the doctors were working on a design for a prosthetic leg that would bend at the knee and function much like a normal leg. To do this, they felt it would be necessary to amputate my right foot in order for the knee joint to be in the proper position. As far as my parents and I were concerned, this was *not* an option. This idea, *if* it worked, would enable me to walk. However, I would lose the ability to accomplish all the things I was already doing with that foot. Therefore, while plans for an alternative prosthetic leg were being made, I returned home to begin fourth grade at West End.

I returned to Kessler for a month in December to learn to use the new prosthetic leg. During this trip, I was so homesick that my weekly Sunday phone calls with Mom and Dad only made matters worse. This was far different from my first visit in large part because of the time of year I was there. Just hearing the sound of my parents voices caused me to get choked up to the point that I could hardly speak. In an effort to make things better, one of the nurses took me to her home over the holidays. I appreciated her kindness, but my tenth birthday and Christmas celebrations were just not the same.

The new custom-made artificial leg failed to be beneficial. Unfortunately, due to my underdeveloped and dislocated hips, this prosthesis caused me a lot of discomfort and pain, proving to be more harmful than helpful. In addition, this option wasn't very practical in that my feet were not free to be "my hands" when I needed them. This was also true of the leg brace that I had been using.

Although my visits to Kessler were not making strides with the walking apparatus, one particular therapy was proving very beneficial for me. Because of my cleft palate, my speech had a nasal tone and I incorrectly pronounced my words. This was especially true when I was nervous or excited. Thanks to speech therapy my communication skills greatly improved.

CHAPTER 6

Valley of Miracles

*I lift up my eyes to the hills – where does my help
come from? My help comes from the Lord, the
maker of heaven and earth.
Psalm 121:1–2*

At the beginning of each West End school year, several of my handicapped schoolmates shared stories of their overnight summer camp experiences. Their stories intrigued me so much that I began to personally consider this option. The following summer, after going through the necessary application procedures, I was excited to hear that I had been accepted to attend.

Camp Easter Seal is a summer camp for handicapped children located in Craig County about thirty-five miles northwest of my hometown. It's a beautiful and peaceful valley surrounded by mountains on one side and a bubbling, cool, clear creek on the other. All around is the smell of evergreens, and plenty of fresh country air.

Children with every type of physical and mental disability are eligible to attend Camp Easter Seal. The staff is highly qualified to assist each camper while encouraging them to reach their highest potential. It is a place where children who are "different" in the normal world, don't *feel* different. At camp, they are accepted in every way. While learning some of life's lessons, the campers are challenged to become as independent as possible.

At the time I attended, there were three camp sessions offered, each lasting three weeks. I was happy to be chosen to attend the first session, and eager to become a part of this camping experience.

Upon arrival, each child is assigned to a cabin containing several bunk beds, and daily activities are scheduled for each cabin on a rotating basis. I enthusiastically participated in such things as swimming, Arts and Crafts, cookouts, overnight camping, horseback riding, and nature hikes. In addition, my fellow campers and I took long strolls or *rolls* around the camp grounds picking daisies, looking for four-leaf clovers, and chasing frogs. Another especially fun thing for me was playing on specially designed swings made for those who could not hold on. Because of my unique way of doing things, I was given the nicknames Thumbs and Twinkle Toes.

Camp Easter Seal was often referred to as the "Valley of Miracles" because of the many first time accomplishments that took place there. Some learned to correctly pronounce words, some learned to swim or ride a horse, and some even walked for the first time. Whenever this occurred, a celebration with recognition and praise took place at mealtime in the dining hall.

The overall experience at camp really gave me a new level of self-confidence. There wasn't anything that I wouldn't try. You should have seen my mom's facial expression the first time she saw me dive off the diving board. Of course, she knew I could swim, but I'm sure she thought I'd really "gone off the deep end" this time. She often said, "I'm not surprised at anything Norma does, especially if she puts her mind to it."

I loved everything about being at camp. Consequently, at the end of my three week stay, I was extremely sad about leaving, and asked if it would be possible to stay another session. Unfortunately, the spots were filled until the last session, so I quickly signed up to return then. These plans allowed me to spend two-thirds of that summer at camp. I was thrilled!

The following summer, I eagerly applied in advance for all three sessions. I soon became actively involved, and one of the most enthusiastic participants. In fact, I enjoyed it so much that after turning sixteen I took a position as one of the camp counselors and was so proud to have a real summer job. The campers assigned to me were fairly self-sufficient; nonetheless, I took my responsibility for them seriously. As I gained more experience and confidence, I was made an assistant to the arts and crafts director. After serving as an assistant for nine years, I was promoted to the director position, which I held for two subsequent years. This was a great fit for me as I enjoyed the challenge of planning creative activities, and thoroughly enjoyed working with all the kids and sharing in their accomplishments.

One of my fondest memories of teaching involved a little girl with Down's syndrome. We were making beanie caps that day, and I told the children to watch me and then do exactly as I was showing them. When each child began to make his or her beanie, I noticed a special little girl had taken my instructions quite literally. She had taken off her shoes and was trying to make the beanie with her toes "just like" her instructor.

Another cherished memory involved hiking with campers and counselors up the mountain, located behind the campsite. One particular summer, it was my turn to "climb" this mountain. I was elated when several of the strong male counselors volunteered to take turns carrying me up a few yards at a time until we reached the top. What made this event even more special was spending the night up there, and watching a full moon come over the ridge. It truly was a beautiful mountain-top experience. When morning came, so did a summer shower which caught us completely by surprise. Of course, we had no rain gear. As we were preparing to return to camp, there was nothing for us to do but make a run for it down the hillside—everyone that is, but me. My friends' quick thinking resulted in cutting leg holes in a duffle bag. They placed me feet first in the bag, tied a rope around my waist, and held it tightly as I slid down the mountainside. Although I experienced a rather bumpy ride, we all returned to camp soaking wet, covered in mud, and laughing hysterically.

Although most of the times at camp were fun, I also had my share of bumps and bruises. For instance, I had a few bloody noses from catching my wheelchair in a heavy door, as I tried to push my way through. I made it, but my chair didn't, ouch! Another time, a flaming marshmallow was dropped on my foot, resulting in a second-degree burn. My most traumatic accident resulted from clowning around while sitting on a counselor's lap in my wheelchair. Another counselor proceeded to push us rather fast when my wheelchair ran off the sidewalk, throwing me headfirst into the grass. I was rushed to a hospital about thirty-five miles away. They say I kept repeating *where's my shoe?* the entire trip. I woke up later in my own bed at home, and my parents explained that I had suffered a concussion. They never knew what to expect next.

Aside from all the fun and friendships I had at camp, I also learned how to be self-sufficient. One of the occupational therapists, my friend Lola, showed me various ways to accomplish great feats. By using a bath brush attached to an extension, I could successfully bathe myself. I also learned to shampoo my hair by using a hairbrush. I have Lola to thank for all these things. Another accomplishment on my road to independence involved what I call the "toilet thingy." It was a folding apparatus that allowed me to go to the bathroom independently. At one end was a clothespin that held the toilet paper in place. At the other end was a mouth piece made from a personalized dental impression allowing for a firmer grip and better control.

On August 1, 1969, at three thirty-four in the afternoon, I buttoned my first button by using a special stick with a hook on the end. This gave me such confidence that I attempted to dress myself without any assistance. I cried happy tears at my success in accomplishing this, even though it took me an hour and a half.

By the end of that summer, at the age of twenty-four there was very little that I could not do for myself. It was at Camp Easter Seal that I gained an overwhelming sense of self-confidence and hope which gave flight to my natural-born independent spirit.

CHAPTER 7

Teamwork Brings Honors

*Because you are my help, I sing in the shadow
of your wings. My soul clings to you;
your right hand upholds me.
Psalm 63:7–8*

Jefferson High School was typical of most schools during the sixties—three stories high with lots of stairs and no elevators or ramps—not at all accessible for someone in a wheelchair. But I had my mind set on returning to public school. I could still ride the handicap bus, so transportation would not be a problem. The school authorities were reluctant, but with my parents' support they agreed to let me give it a try. Once again, the only accommodation I would need was a desktop placed on the floor of each of my classrooms.

I made lots of friends at Jefferson; and there was always someone eager to help when I needed to pack or unpack my books, sharpen a pencil, or even "raise a hand." Usually, several of my girlfriends accompanied me from class to class with much giggling and chatting. I was always included in conversations about the latest hairstyles and clothes fads as well as conversations about guys.

Speaking of guys, the football team volunteered to carry me in my wheelchair up and down the stairs when needed. Their reward was being excused from their classes five minutes early. I became the envy of most of the girls at Jefferson, and of course *foot*ball quickly became my favorite sport. I got to know the players quite well and demonstrated my appreciation for their strong arms of support by rooting for them from the stands at every Friday night home game. Subsequently, I learned a lot about football. I became one of their most loyal and enthusiastic fans, not to mention one of the loudest.

There are many fond memories of my high school days; but when it came to academics, I set very high standards for myself. I studied diligently, and wanted to make good grades. I suppose I wanted to prove to myself and others that I could succeed scholastically.

Typing and shorthand were two of my favorite subjects. It wasn't that I had a mind for business—I'm more of a "people person"—but I enjoy a challenge, and typing with my toes was certainly that. I used my toes to open a folder, select a single sheet of paper, and insert the paper into the typewriter (obviously before the computer age). Shorthand was also fascinating to me, and was useful in taking lecture notes.

As the local newspapers somehow heard about my story, they were curious and wanted to know more. Several interviews and articles followed, and by my senior year, I had become quite the hometown celebrity. There were headlines that read, "Courage takes the Place of Arms," "Armless Girl Leads Normal Life"; and the articles explained how *normal* and well adjusted my life seemed to be. They included pictures of me typing, the football players carrying me in my wheelchair down the stairs, and hanging out with my girlfriends between classes. I never suffered from lack of attention, and loved every minute of it.

During my junior year, I applied to become a member of the National Honor Society which recognized students of high character, service, and scholastic achievement. A 4.0 average and faculty approval were required for membership.

The event took place in the school auditorium, and no one knew beforehand who would be selected. It was an exciting and thrilling moment as my classmates and I awaited the names to be announced. When my name was called, I was surprised and honored to be tapped into this elite group of students by one of my best friends, Ellen.

TEAMWORK BRINGS HONORS

During my high school years, I received other honors and recognitions. I was awarded the Daughters of the American Revolution Good Citizen Award for scholastic achievements, and I and one of my football player friends, were voted the Friendliest in the senior class. I was also among the chosen of Jefferson's top seniors to be honored at a banquet where Virginia Delegate M. Caldwell Butler was the guest speaker. The values, excellence, independence, and responsibilities instilled in me by my parents and teachers were reaping rewards far greater than ever expected.

When commencement day on June 7, 1963 arrived, and my name was called to receive my high school diploma, the entire student body stood and applauded. I was suddenly overcome with mixed emotions. I cried tears of joy that God had given me such determination and desire to succeed, and I cried tears of sadness at leaving many who had become so dear to me. I graduated eleventh in a class of 220 students, and always felt that if I had tried just a little harder, I could have been in the top ten. Ugh!

Chapter 8

Seeking New Heights

*I can do everything through him
who gives me strength.
Philippians 4:13*

When I completed high school, many of the graduates went to work at local businesses or joined the military service. College was encouraged, but was not a natural expectation. Most of my friends had plans to attend college, so naturally I wanted to experience this as well. I applied to Roanoke College, one of the local schools, and also visited the University of Illinois Southern campus. UISC was one of the few colleges with special provisions for handicapped students. The campus and the academic program were quite impressive. Although I did not have my heart set on attending there, it was disappointing when I failed to meet their required level of independence for acceptance.

I was accepted at Roanoke College, but really wanted to attend a school outside of my home town, largely because of my ambition to test my independence. Since I had not yet chosen my major, I decided to take the basic required classes locally at the University of Virginia, Roanoke Extension. This would give me more time to consider other educational options.

The UVA extension was located in a large old stately house, with some classes meeting in an adjacent carriage house. There were many steps in the main building; therefore, I had to be carried in my wheelchair up and down some narrow stairways. This brought back some fond memories of my high school days. Once again, several strong, able-bodied male students were willing to lend a hand. You didn't hear me complain.

I completed a variety of general subjects such as English, math, history, and economics. I also took a psychology course which proved quite interesting to me, and seemed to confirm my desire to work with people. What I really wanted to do was become an occupational or speech therapist, but neither option seemed practical for me because of my physical limitations. So after completing two years at the extension, with still no clear direction for a degree, I decided to take a job at the Easter Seal Society state headquarters in Roanoke. It was an easy transition, since I was still working at the camp during the summer months and already knew many of the workers there.

Although I was assigned to work in the mailroom, my first year involved a lot of public relations work which I thoroughly enjoyed. I traveled with area representatives throughout Virginia, relating stories and information about the Easter Seal Society's work with disabled children and adults, particularly the children's camping program. As part of the program, I sang and played my electric chord organ for various charitable organizations. I'm not sure they were as impressed with my singing as with my ability to play the organ with my feet.

Since I love to sing and talk with people, this PR job seemed an ideal one for me. My gift of gab seemed to help others feel more comfortable around me, and I can't say I've ever met a stranger. As the PR work subsided, however, I spent more of my time working as a file clerk in the mailroom of Easter Seal's home office. My job there was keeping address labels up to date with current telephone directories throughout the state. For almost three years, I flipped through thousands of metal addressograph plates with the toes of my right foot to check their accuracy. At the same time, I held a pencil in my left foot marking through names and addresses as each was completed. This task, although necessary, was not very satisfying to me. It was without a doubt the most tedious, repetitive, and boring job I've ever had.

But the people there were good to me, and I did continue to work at the camp during the summer months.

When I returned to camp in the summer of 1967, I began to talk with fellow staff members about the career possibilities in my future. One of my close counselor friends suggested that I consider returning to school. Lizz was a student at Emory & Henry College, a small church-sponsored school in southwest Virginia. The campus layout was not especially disability accessible, but as she described its warm and friendly atmosphere, the idea became quite alluring to me.

One night, after all the campers were safely tucked into their bunks and the counselors had collapsed from exhaustion, Lizz and I sat up much of the night talking, and composing a letter to the Dean of Women at E&H requesting that they consider my application for admission. Now, all we could do was pray and wait. After camp was over, I returned to my mailroom job while teaching the Young Adult Sunday School class, and singing in the choir at my home church.

After several weeks, an E&H application arrived in my mailbox. I was extremely excited about this opportunity and promptly completed and submitted all the necessary forms. Then there was more waiting, which is not an easy thing for me. Although hoping for the best, I was somewhat trying to protect myself from any possible disappointment. In the meantime, my parents and I received a letter signed by twenty girls of the Martha Washington dormitory at Emory & Henry, stating their commitment and pledge to help and support me on campus. Lizz had told them about my desire to attend college which prompted them to speak to the Dean of Women on my behalf. All this provided great encouragement as I eagerly awaited news from the Admissions Office.

CHAPTER 9
Persistence Paves the Way

*You need to persevere so that when you have done the will of God,
you will receive what he has promised.*
Hebrews 10:36

The Board of Admissions, after carefully considering my application invited my parents and me to visit Emory & Henry College. The campus was small and beautiful, but quite hilly, with stairs in most of the buildings. In our meeting with the admissions board, it was difficult to read the thoughts of those present, with the exception of the Dean of Women. She felt the girls who offered their help were sincere, but was concerned there would be times they would not be available. I must admit, I was having similar doubts and fears myself. The thought of taking notes in class, keeping up with assignments, typing reports and term papers, taking exams—all the usual academic pressures—was quite scary. Facing these tasks would be challenging enough, but I would face the added responsibility of arranging for my personal care and getting to and from classes, the library, the cafeteria, and the chapel.

Leaving the security I had at home and work was admittedly a bit frightening, but I've always told others, "You'll never know if you don't try." It was time to practice what I preached. I find new adventures exciting, but this would be the greatest one yet. It was important for me to try my wings, and discover my potential for independence. All I wanted was for the admission's board to allow me that opportunity. If it became too difficult, I assured them that I would be the first to admit it, and would bow out graciously.

After what seemed like a very long time, I received a letter in my mailbox from E&H. With great anticipation, I opened the letter and was extremely pleased to learn that I had been accepted. I could not wait for the arrival of my first college day; however, there was much to do to prepare for that time.

The day finally arrived to settle in on campus. I watched my parents unpack our fully loaded station wagon, and we all met many of the girls who had written encouraging letters to us. They were quite friendly and went out of their way to make this big step in my life as easy as possible. As I said goodbye to Mom and Dad, and watched them drive away, mixed emotions brought tears to my eyes. Soon after, I made the decision not to go home for a visit until Thanksgiving break; otherwise, I might be tempted not to return.

I was assigned a room in the Martha Washington dormitory, known as MaWa, the only dorm on campus with an elevator. It didn't take long to get to know my roommate and the other girls on the third floor west wing. They proved sincere in their eagerness to make me feel welcome and comfortable. There was always someone around when I needed assistance, or just a listening ear. I was never shy about asking for things I really needed, but never wanted to be a burden. For that reason, I made a decision early on to change roommates each year. Getting to classes wasn't the problem I had anticipated. After all, Emory & Henry had lots of handsome coeds around to carry me in my wheelchair up and down the stairs. And one campus fraternity volunteered to be on call, particularly when the weather was bad and I needed a ride.

Most of the girls on my hall belonged to a sorority, which happened to be the sister sorority of my "adopted" fraternity brothers. I wanted to become an official sister to these girls who had devoted their time to me, but the process would not be easy. This required a lot of time, and I wasn't sure I could handle the extra stress and keep up with my studies. I decided to give it a try, and after a couple weeks of hard rushing, I was accepted into the sorority. I was so happy to be a part of this sisterhood. We became close friends, and shared many special times together.

It was only natural for me to pursue music education in college. As I mentioned earlier, I sang in the church choir, and as a little girl, Dad always insisted that I sing and play my chord organ for our house guests. I learned to read music when I took piano lessons from one of my teachers at West End Elementary. Although music and singing had always been a part of my life, I had not received any formal voice lessons until my days at E&H.

Singing in the choir was my favorite and most memorable college activity. We were privileged to have one of the best chorus directors around. Not only was he a good director, but Doc, as we called him, was also a positive Christian role model who always inspired our best performance. Each year, I sang in the chapel choir, and ambitiously auditioned for the concert choir. The concert choir routinely went on a spring tour, mostly traveling on the East Coast with an occasional trip to a foreign country. Because Doc was very particular in choosing this select group, you cannot imagine how overjoyed I was to finally be chosen as a member for my senior year.

Throughout my year in concert choir, we held many performances locally and statewide. For our spring tour, we traveled to New Orleans in a chartered bus. Our time together was so much fun, filled with sounds of song and laughter. Concerts were planned to take place in churches along the way, and we often stayed in pairs or small groups in church members' homes overnight. Prior to arriving in New Orleans, Doc had warned us that our time for sight-seeing would be limited. There were two concerts the following day and getting the necessary rest to perform well was Doc's primary concern. None of us wanted to let him down, but at the same time, we wanted to experience New Orleans. Thankfully, we managed to take in most of the sites and activities on Bourbon Street, as well as perform beyond our greatest expectations for both concerts. Doc was more than pleased, and the satisfaction we all felt with this accomplishment was overwhelming.

My college days were not easy, but quite rewarding and fulfilling. There were many late nights with little sleep. The days were filled with classes, studying, sorority meetings, choir rehearsals, and of course room to room visiting in the dorm. There were also strolls around campus, to the post office for letters or packages from home, and visits to the popular duck pond. There are so many fond memories of my days at Emory & Henry. After three years, I graduated with an interdisciplinary major in sociology, psychology, and history, with a minor degree in music. I am so grateful for the entire experience of campus life. Graduation was held outside on a beautiful spring day. As my name was called to receive my diploma, I was especially touched when the crowd gave a standing ovation in my honor. The tears I shed that day were an outward expression of the satisfaction I felt from reaching a new level of independence in my life.

CHAPTER 10

Feet at Work

For it is God who works in you to will and to act according to his good purpose.
Philippians 2:13

I was glad to be home after graduation, and away from the pressures of college life. It was a welcome change to return to my work at Camp Easter Seal that summer. As for future employment, I would seek information and advice through my contacts at camp. Thankfully, I had a job for the summer and just *maybe* my future would become clearer as the summer went by. Mickey, a coworker at camp, who also worked at the Easter Seal home office, happened to be a member of the Mayor's Committee for Employment of the Handicapped. During one of our conversations, he asked if I had ever considered working at the Veterans Administration Hospital. This question came as a surprise. The only previous contact I had with the VA involved the making of my toilet assistance apparatus, but I was certainly willing to pursue the possibility. Mickey had far more knowledge and influence concerning work at the VA Hospital than I realized. Before I knew it, I was being interviewed by the chief and several other respected staff members of the Psychology Department. I was a nervous wreck! Although I knew very little about vocational counseling, I was offered a job as a specialist which fortunately included on-the-job training. This new career opportunity came sooner than I ever expected.

I finished my summer at camp and started in my new job only two days later. Although I loved my job at camp, it required constant availability to assist in the needs of others. The excitement of graduation combined with the physical and emotional strain at camp had taken its toll on me. Fortunately, the chief of the Psychology Service recognized my symptoms, and recommended that I see the staff doctor. Exhaustion had set in. Subsequently, I was sent home to rest the remainder of my first week.

Upon my return to work, I discovered there was a lot to learn. I would work with physically and/or psychiatrically disabled veterans with identified adjustment problems resulting most often from their military experiences. They were referred to me for help in preparing to return to civilian life after an extended stay in the hospital.

My office was set up to suit my needs and had several unique features. The first was a low doorknob for my convenience. Then there was the beautiful double drawer desk which was specially made for me in the hospital woodshop. It stood twelve inches off the floor, an ideal height for writing patient reports. The telephone was placed where I could pick up the receiver between my chin and shoulder, freeing my feet for dialing or taking notes. My child-size motorized wheelchair enabled me access to any area of the large hospital grounds without assistance. Even the Psychology Service restroom was modified so that I could use it independently.

I usually held several counseling sessions with each in-hospital client, administering various interest and personality tests to determine a realistic vocational objective. Then there was the difficult task of matching job capabilities with available positions. This usually required phoning various employers, or scheduling the veteran with the state employment commission for job interviews. Once a veteran was discharged from the hospital, it was difficult to follow his or her progress. Unfortunately, the ones we most often saw were the ones who were readmitted. But occasionally, someone would return just to say thanks. Those were the ones who made it all worthwhile.

In addition to my vocational counseling responsibilities, I also enjoyed working with recovering alcoholics as a group facilitator. Many of these patients were not there because they wanted to be, and some were eager to blame anyone but themselves for their predicament. I was quick to point out that some things in life are neither fair nor fixable, but would not allow the poor-pitiful-me attitude to prevail. Our discussions centered around how best to react to the circumstances in our lives. We can develop a negative attitude and become a victim, or have a positive outlook and become victorious. In my own life, I've considered most obstacles as a challenge to try even harder.

I was often told that I worked well with disabled veterans, particularly those who suffered from depression. My physical presence seemed to give them encouragement in a unique way which made it difficult for them to say "I can't." Through helping others in their lives, I gained confidence in my own ability to make a difference in the world. Although I knew things were going well at work, I was shocked when in 1974 I was chosen among thirty-seven VA disabled employees to be recognized nationally for excellence in job performance.

In the spring of 1975, my parents and I traveled to Washington DC to participate in the awards festivities. The VA held a reception for me at the national headquarters where they presented me with an official certificate of honor and a United States flag that had flown over the US Capitol Building. Then came the day we had waited for, the day I would officially become the VA's Outstanding Handicapped Federal Employee of the Year. The ceremony took place at the Commerce Building, and the awards—representing ten different federal agencies—were presented by Vice President Nelson D. Rockefeller. After nervously waiting and watching all the other recipients, it was finally my turn to be recognized. I presented to the Vice President a *foot-printed scroll* which I had especially written in calligraphy for him. It contained a quote by Henry Viscardi which read:

A Productive Life

"Neither pensions, parades nor pity can substitute for the sweet dignity of a productive life."

"I seek opportunity — not security. I do not wish to be a kept citizen, humbled and dulled by having the state look after me. I want to take the calculated risk; to dream and to build, to fail and to succeed. I refuse to barter incentive for a dole. I prefer the challenges of life to the guaranteed existence..."

Henry Viscardi

With tears in his eyes, Mr. Rockefeller seemed moved by my thoughtfulness, and kissed me on the cheek. There were many pictures and reports of this momentous occasion. However, most cherished of all were the words my Dad shared with one newspaper reporter, "The doctors said she would never live a 'normal' life. Now look at her. She's a very determined person, and we are proud of all she has done."

As a result of the national award, other awards surprisingly followed. I was named *Woman of the Year* by area chapters of the Beta Sigma Phi Sorority, and presented the 1976 Young Alumnus Award by Emory & Henry College. I was certainly honored to receive these awards, but also felt that I had simply been doing the job that I had been given to do.

Chapter 11

Prisoners Give Freedom

> *Since we are surrounded by such a great cloud of witnesses, let us throw off everything that hinders and the sin that so easily entangles, and let us run with perseverance the race marked out for us.*
> *Hebrews 12:1*

Despite my independence, I still relied on others for transportation. The VA was located close to home, but I had to depend on my parents to get me there. A fellow employee, who lived in my neighborhood, began giving me rides. Although I appreciated his generosity, I still yearned for independence in this area of my life.

My desire to drive had been previously reported in a newspaper article written several years earlier. In that article, I simply stated that "someday I hoped to drive." A group of prison inmates at the Virginia State Penitentiary, who were also members of the prison chapter of Jaycees, was seeking ideas for a humanitarian project. The wife of one of their shop instructors remembered reading the article about me, and shared this information with her husband. They felt it would be a good opportunity for the prisoners to have an effect on someone else's life in a positive way. Therefore, after much discussion "Project Norma" was born.

The plan was to raise enough money to purchase a van, and then personally install it with the needed handicap equipment. In order to raise money for the project, the inmates acquired a cleanup contract to work at the Virginia State Fair. Twenty-seven of the inmates then got approval to leave the prison grounds to participate. They worked very hard for thirty days emptying trash, selling scrap metals and papers, and manning a "Cream the Car" activity, where participants paid to sledge hammer an automobile donated by a local salvage company. Those not allowed to work at the fair took care of the bookkeeping, and corresponding with companies that specialized in handicap driving equipment.

With the money raised at the fair, the Jaycees purchased a van from a local car dealership. Upon realizing they were not trained to make the necessary changes themselves, they sent the van to Drive Master in New Jersey for the specified modifications. Mine would be the first vehicle to be equipped with all foot controls. This would add an additional challenge for the designers. The plan was to place a small disk wheel on the floor of the driver's side to be operated with my left foot. The wheel would contain a knob for holding it and steering the van. After some of the equipment was installed, my parents and I went to New Jersey for fittings and measurements.

At the time this project was going on, I was participating in a graduate work and study program in Richmond. A couple years into my work at the VA, several of my contacts with the Virginia State Rehabilitation Services heightened my interest to pursue a master's degree. Several of these individuals were advancing their education through classes at Virginia Commonwealth University. I had been interested in rehabilitative counseling, and felt this opportunity may open doors for my future. Therefore, I began carpooling with several of the rehab workers attending VCU. Our classes met on Friday evening and Saturday morning, every other weekend. After roughly a year of working full time, keeping up with studies, and traveling to and from Richmond I realized it was too much. Because I was already blessed with a good job, I opted to drop the classes.

My time in Richmond gave me the opportunity to visit the penitentiary several times, allowing me to meet and get to know the guys involved in "Project Norma." This I considered a huge bonus, which otherwise would not have occurred had I not taken classes at VCU. The prisoners, meanwhile, received several awards at the State Jaycee Convention in Roanoke where they were recognized nationally for their efforts.

At the completion of the project, a presentation ceremony was planned to take place on the grounds of the state penitentiary on June 14, 1974. It would take place in the inner courtyard, so that all but maximum security prisoners could be part of the celebration. It was an exciting time for me, a day I had looked forward to for quite a while. I and several of my family members and friends, arrived early as planned, allowing time to test drive the van prior to the actual presentation. For security purposes, the ceremony itself was on a strict schedule. The van, driven from New Jersey by one of the mechanics who installed the special equipment, unfortunately arrived barely in time for the ceremony. I had hoped to have time for a practice run beforehand, but with no time available, things proceeded as scheduled.

I could never have imagined the big production my prison friends had planned for me. A stage had been set up, a band played, and there were hundreds of inmates watching from the stands. Reporters and TV cameras were everywhere. The Jaycees carried banners that read "Keep on Truckin'," "Ride Norma Ride," and "We Love You Norma."

The ceremony began right on schedule. In appreciation for what these guys had done for me, I played "Welcome to my Morning (Farewell Andromeda)" on my chord organ while singing the verses beginning with, "Welcome to my happiness…you made my day…I wouldn't change a thing." After this, one burly inmate dropped to his knees beside me, and sang in his baritone voice "The Impossible Dream." He completely melted my heart as I realized one of my biggest dreams was coming true that very day.

When the keys and title to the van were handed over to me, I felt like a queen. Reporters held microphones, and cameras were flashing as I opened the sliding door using the four toggle switches located on the front right fender. After the lift swung out and lowered to the ground, I rolled myself onto the platform and then manipulated other switches to enter the van. The mechanic, who had transported the van, was seated in the front passenger seat in order to give me the necessary instructions. I secured my wheelchair with a bungee cord, and boosted myself into the seat. After fastening my seatbelt, I turned on the ignition with my left foot and lowered the windows electronically. Everyone cheered and gave me a standing ovation. Then, I invited anyone to hop in who wished to take the first ride with me around the courtyard. To my surprise, many of my Jaycee friends piled in, voluntarily placing their lives in my *feet*. We then circled the field as the crowd waved and cheered us on.

I never dreamed this accomplishment would draw so much attention. It was publicized in several newspapers and magazines, and appeared on the national news. Even my aunt and uncle in California were quite surprised when they saw me on their local channel. I will never forget that day, or those prison inmates who spent countless, unselfish hours to make this possible. Their willing hands along with their kind hearts were being used to provide for me this great gift of independence. I will forever be grateful in remembering this special moment of my life.

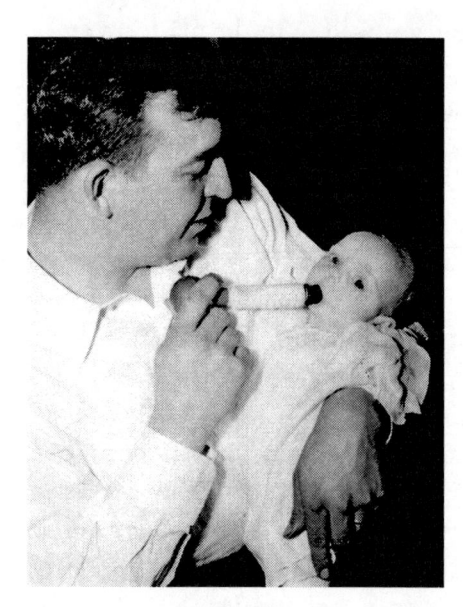

Dad's Creative Baby Bottle

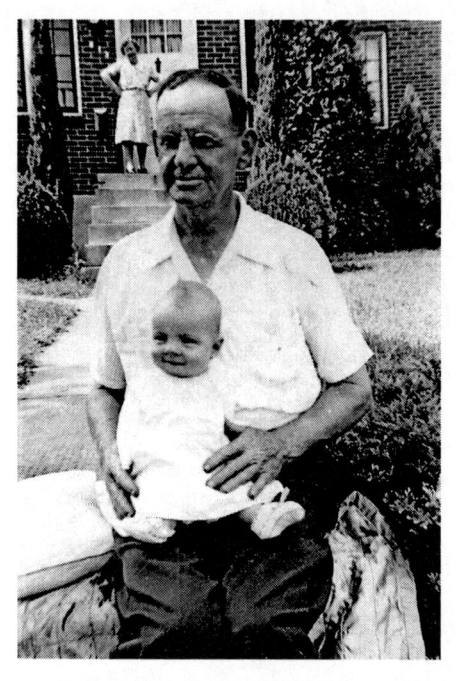

Visit with Granddaddy and Grandma Pritchett

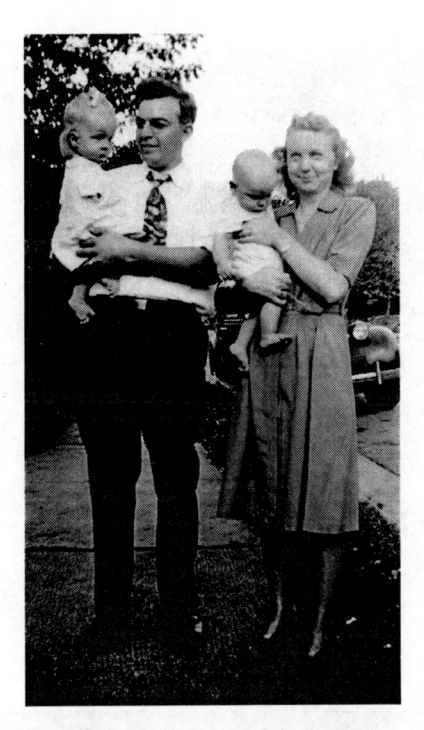

Dad, Mom, me, and Barry

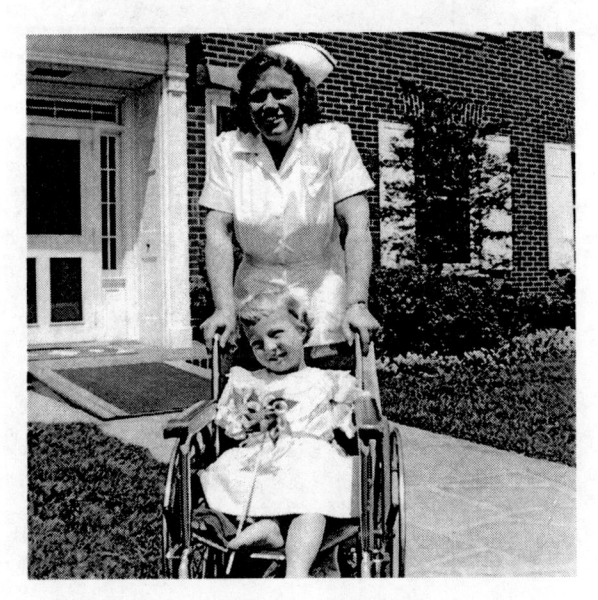

Therapy at Kessler Institute, New Jersey

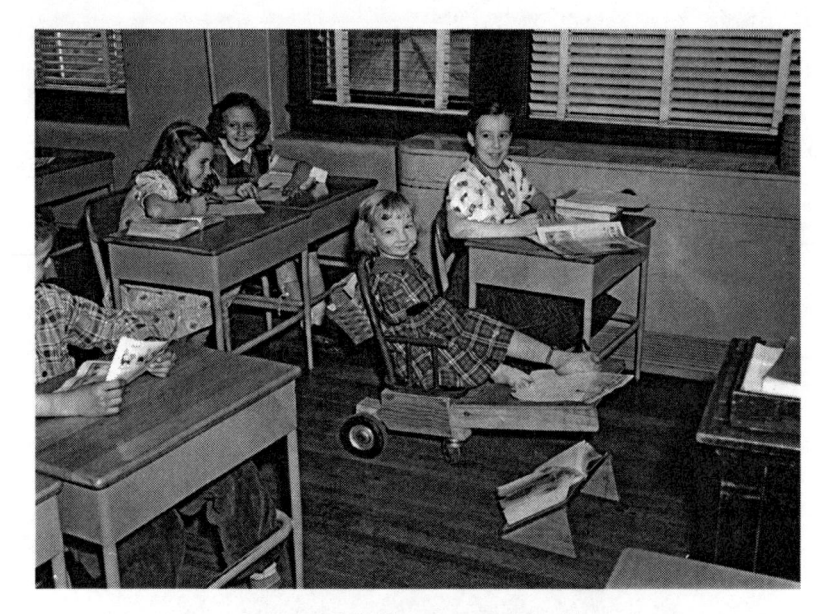

West End Elementary School

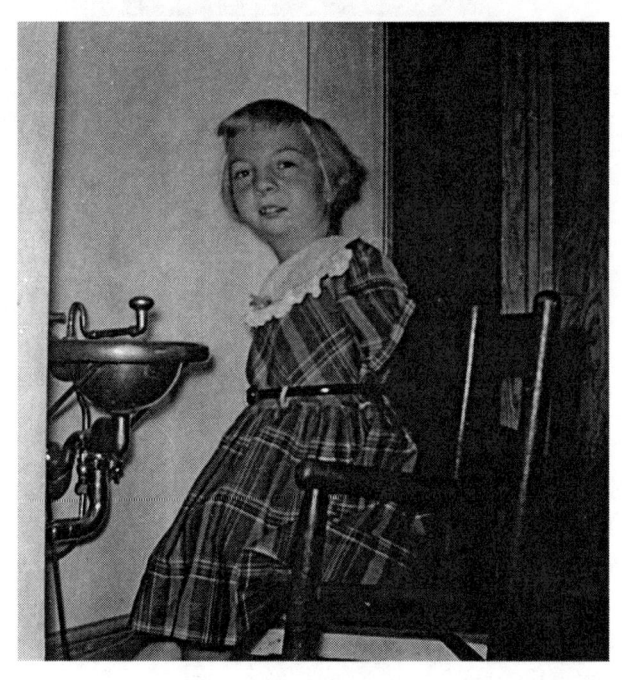

Bedroom Drinking Fountain

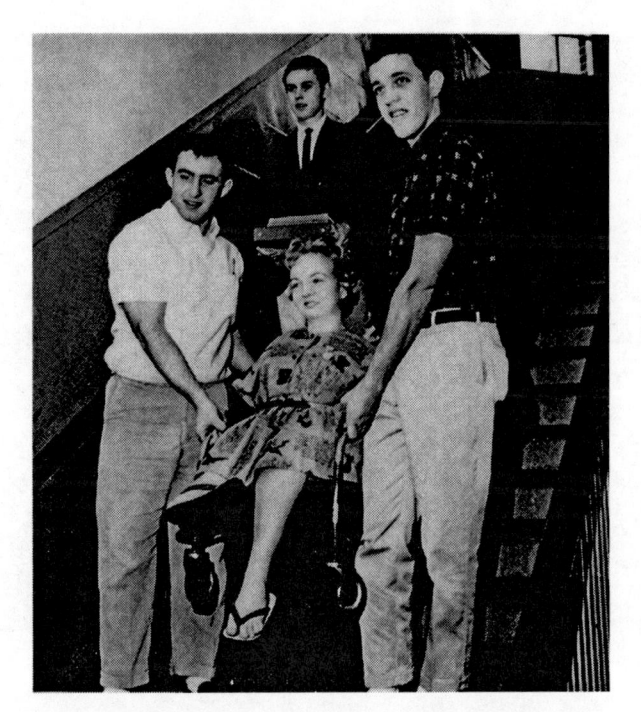

Assistance from High School Football Team

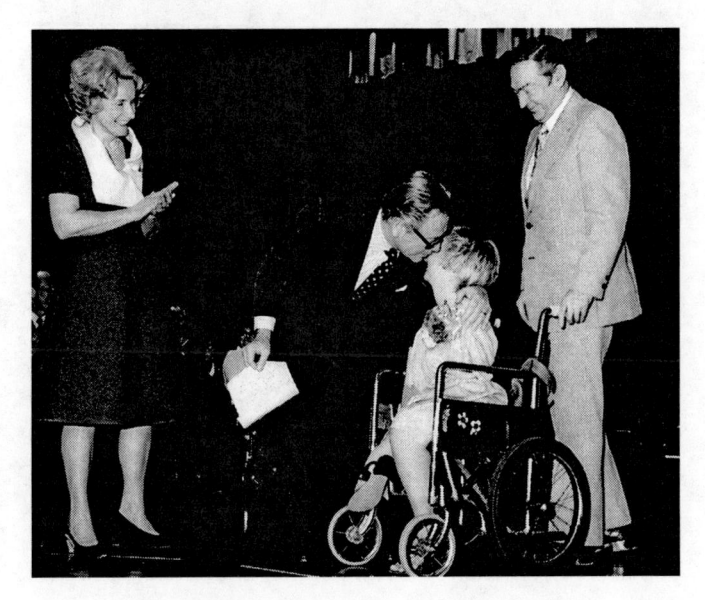

Special Kiss from Vice President Rockefeller

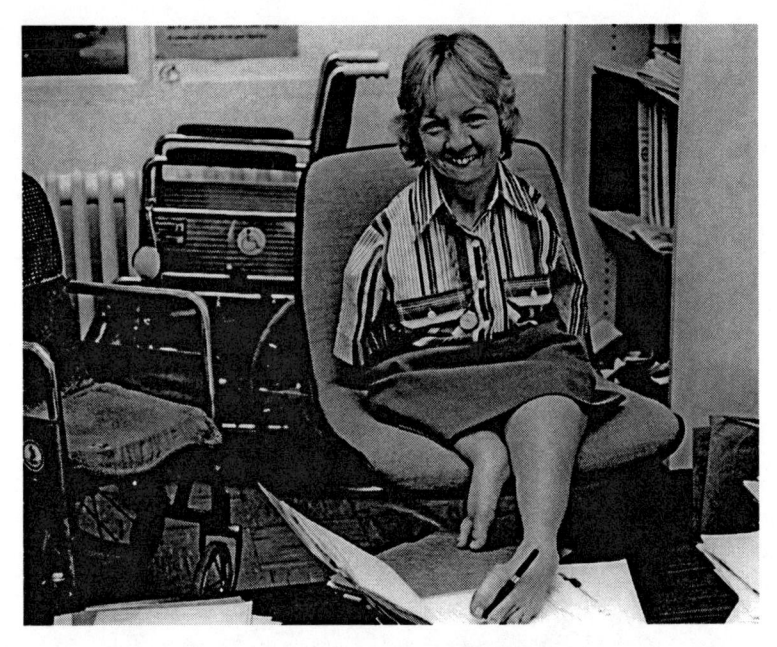

Job at VA Hospital

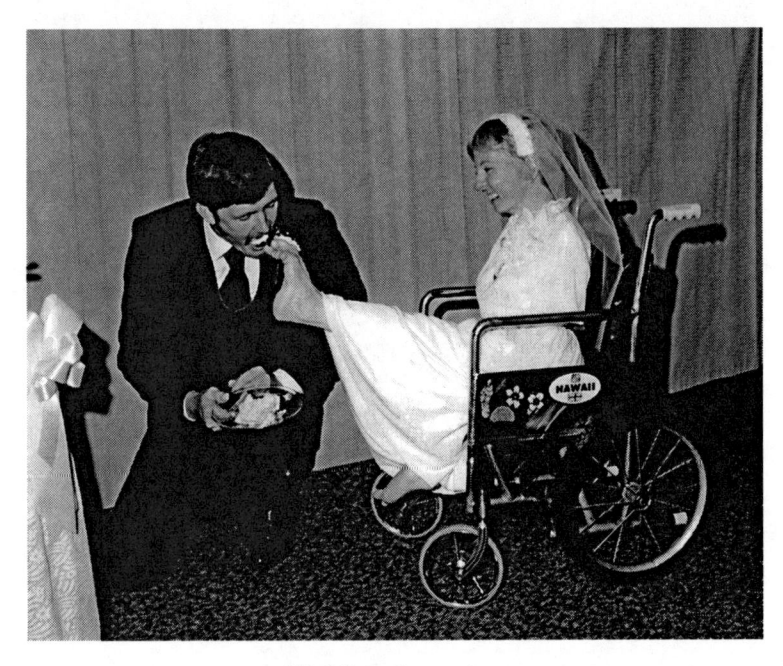

Wedding Reception

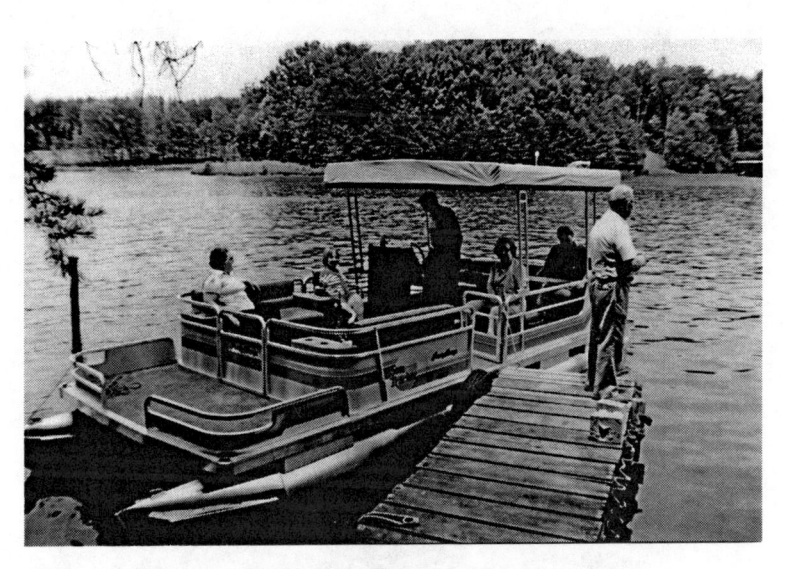

Smith Mountain Lake

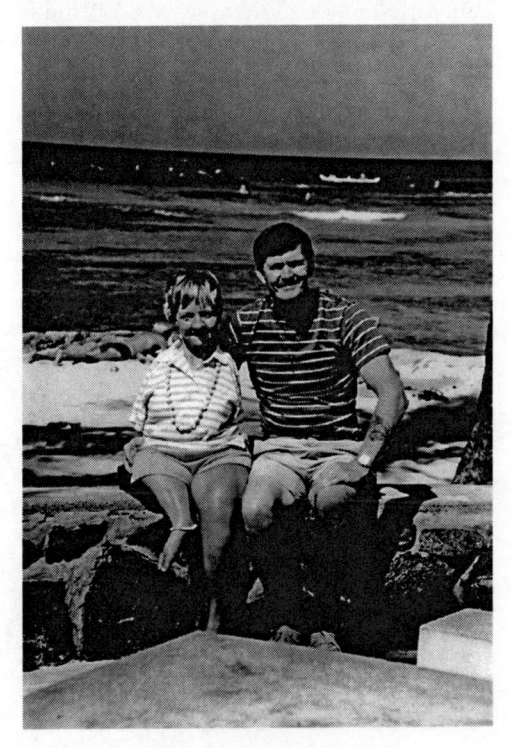

Vacation in Oahu, Hawaii

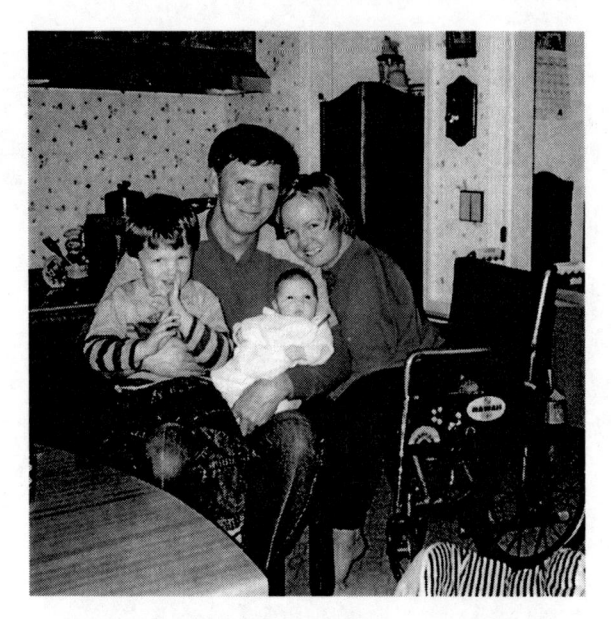

Fun with Grandchildren, Jesse and Brittany

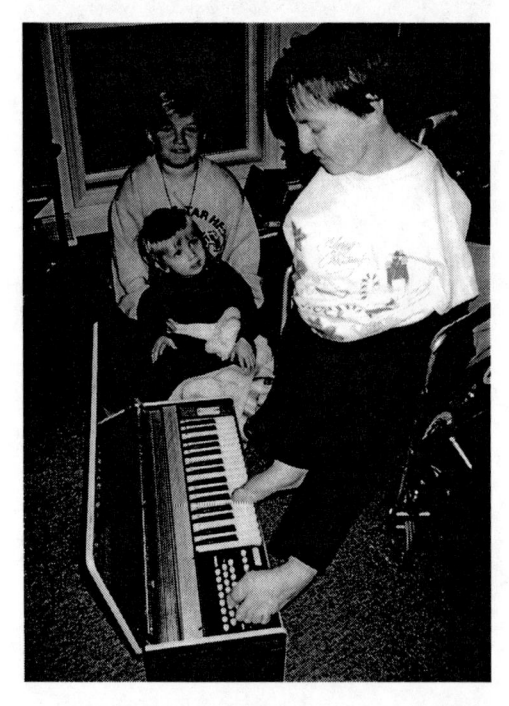

Music with Grandchildren, Jessica and Jeffrey

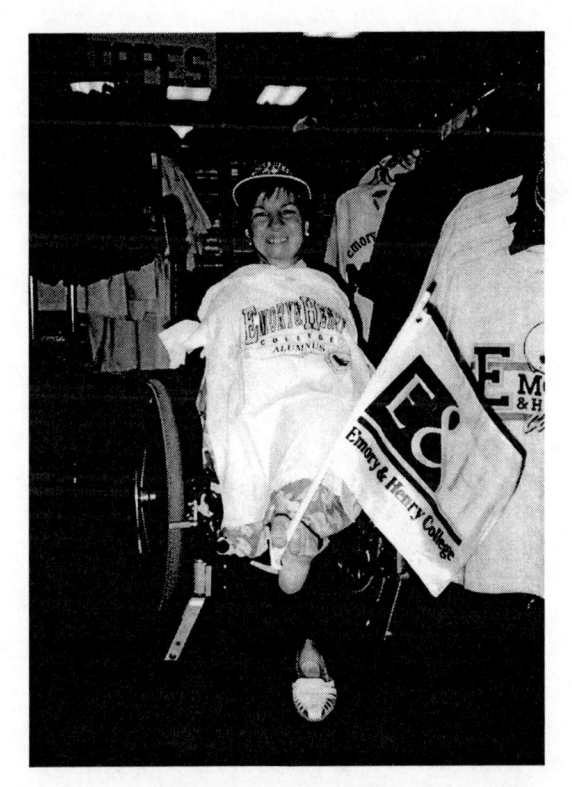

Displaying School Spirit

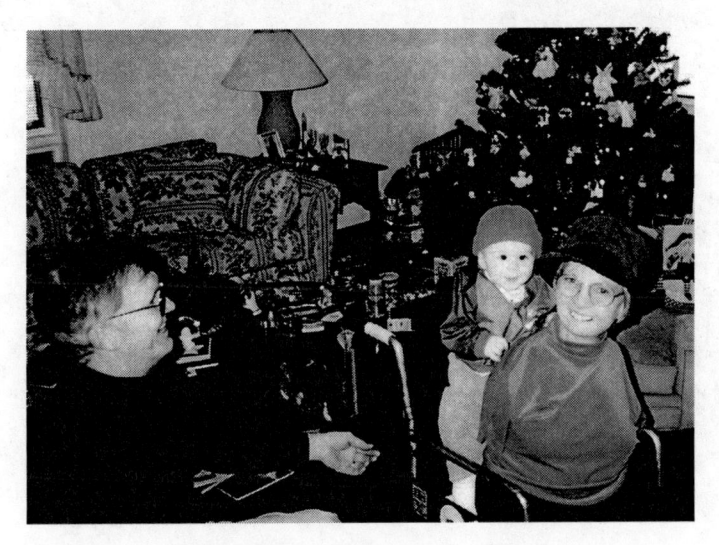

Piggyback with Grandma, Lance

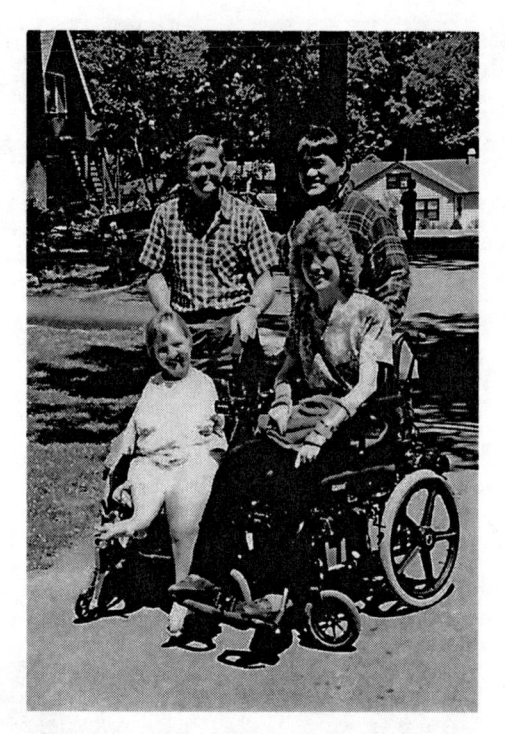

With Ken and Joni Tada at Pocono's Retreat

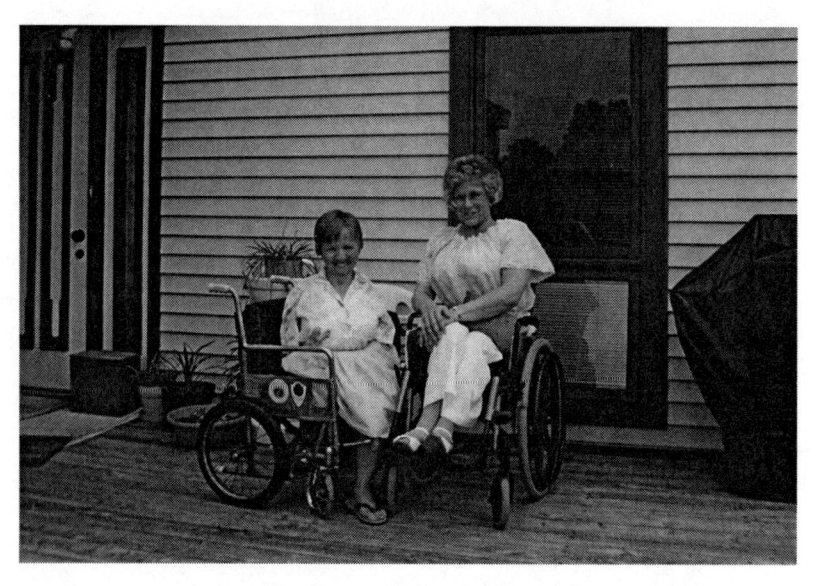

Old School Friend, Joanna

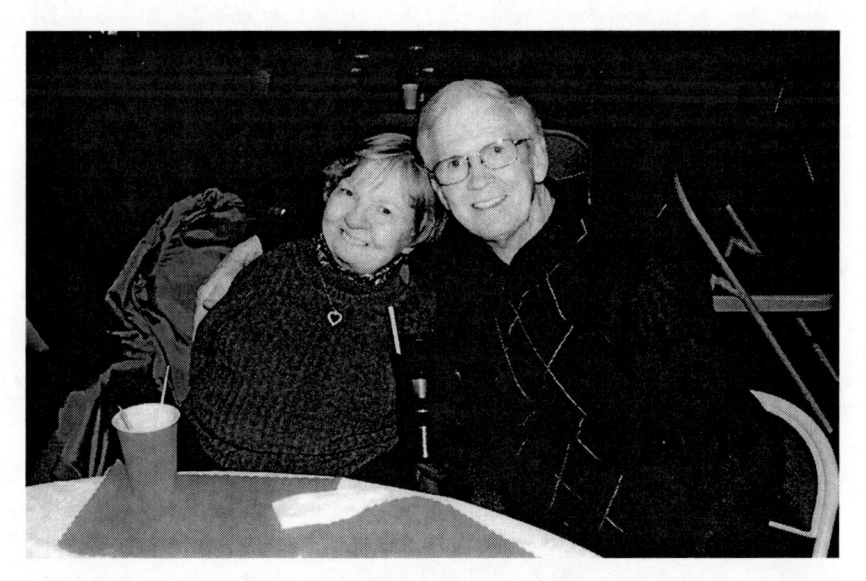

Church Valentine's Dinner

CHAPTER 12

My Father's Hands

*Make it your ambition to lead a quiet life,
to mind your own business and to work with your
hands..., so that your daily life may
win the respect of outsiders.*
1 Thessalonians 4:11–12

I had taken the written test to receive my learner's permit, but of course, I was anxious to get behind the wheel and learn to drive. My first opportunity happened to fall on Father's Day. Dad suggested that we take the van to a nearby school parking lot. He drove there, and I practiced on the school driving range until we were both comfortable with my ability to handle the vehicle. That very day, Dad was so confident in my skills that he encouraged me to drive home. This became a daily practice as we ventured a little further on the main roads each day. Consequently, after only two weeks of "Dad training," my father felt that I was ready to take the driver's test for my license.

When we arrived at the Division of Motor Vehicles, all eyes seemed to find me, and we could only imagine what people were thinking. The employees were having a hard time believing that I had already received my learner's permit. Two attending officers went with me for my road test, which was highly unusual. Because I was not the typical applicant, Dad and I surmised that they felt the need for a second witness. I passed the road test, and was thrilled and excited when they took my picture and issued me my driver's license. No one was prouder than my dad. This accomplishment was so much more meaningful to me due to his involvement, and all the experiences we shared preparing for this day.

So many memorable things happened in my life during the seventies—graduating from college, getting a job with the Veterans Administration, learning to drive, and receiving national recognition for my accomplishments. Things seemed to be going my way. At this point in time, I felt I could do anything I set my mind to. I even began wondering if someday I might be able to live independently.

When I discussed with my parents my thoughts about independent living arrangements, they were reluctant, but willing to help me explore the possibilities. We talked about all the logistics involved, and decided to choose a realtor who could show us homes that might meet my needs. After several viewings, we found there were no suitable homes readily available. Major modifications requiring added expense would have to be made. This was very discouraging. Consequently, we began thinking about designing a single level floor plan ourselves.

Meanwhile, we located two lots each containing a quarter acre of land not far from my job site. Excited about this opportunity, I was ready to purchase one of these properties with visions of future development. My first choice was the more level corner lot, but we were told it was already under contract. While considering the purchase of the other lot, the realtor contacted us to let us know that our original choice was now available. I could hardly contain myself at the thought of having my future home built on this spot.

Not long before that time, Dad had helped my brother, Barry, build his house. Following this experience, Dad believed that he could construct a house to my specifications. He would soon be retiring from the railroad and we all knew Dad's hands couldn't be idle for any length of time.

I was so pleased that Dad wanted to build a house for me. Excitement peaked as we looked at various floor plans and considered features for a low-maintenance dwelling. The one-floor plan we selected had five rooms with two baths, and an attached double garage. The rooms and closets were large enough to allow easy access in a wheelchair. We did make a few changes from the original design, widening the doors, and eliminating all steps. We also selected large double-pane windows with blinds encased between the panes. I especially liked the ability to open and close the bottom portion of the windows by cranking a lever with my foot.

The construction began in early 1978. Barry, other family members and friends joined in and helped along the way. Mom played a special behind-the-scenes role providing meals, drinks and snacks which fueled and sustained everyone during the long hours of work each day. Both my parents endured and sacrificed a lot for my sake—Dad even lost a noticeable amount of weight in the process.

A lot of thought went into selecting each appliance and fixture. The kitchen sink, stovetop, and counters were placed eighteen inches above the floor allowing me easy access from my wheelchair. The built-in oven with front control knobs was installed at an appropriate level along with a small refrigerator, and apartment-size dishwasher. I chose a small upright freezer and a front-loading stackable washer and dryer, to be placed side by side in the utility room located next to the kitchen.

We special ordered a small square bathtub for the master bath. Dad made a padded platform to allow me to safely transfer in and out of the tub. Throughout the house, doorknobs and light switches were placed slightly lower for easy reach. Dad also added an intercom system and electronic locks on outside doors for added security.

After eighteen months of hard work and steady commitment, my dream home was completed and I moved in on June 1, 1979. This new chapter of my life was thrilling, but soon the reality of living independently caused some feelings of anxiousness. Although the house was designed so that I could manage mostly on my own, I felt it would be beneficial to have someone else around for any possible need that might arise as well as for companionship.

While attending a local Christian coffeehouse, I met a girl who was interested in moving out of her parents' home. After becoming more acquainted, we decided to become housemates. I was able to cook, wash dishes, wash clothes, and dust. I also could press my clothes as long as I used a light weight iron and a tabletop ironing board placed on the floor. On the other hand, using the central vacuum proved too difficult. Once attempting this task, I ended up tangled in the long hose and trapped in the corner of the room wishing that someone would come to my rescue. Vacuuming would definitely go on my housemate's to-do list.

My new home was such a special gift that I decided to hold a dedication service roughly a month after moving in. During the service, we asked the blessing of God on this new home and all who entered. My family's minister led the event and one of my cousins closed by singing "Bless this House." There were approximately a hundred people in attendance, including all those who had contributed in some way. This gave me the perfect opportunity to express my gratitude to everyone who had a hand in making this day possible.

CHAPTER 13

Milkshake Made in Heaven

*No eye has seen, no ear has heard,
no mind has conceived what God has prepared
for those who love him.*
1 Corinthians 2:9

Working a full-time job and trying to keep up household chores was all new to me—and no easy task. My housemate was some help, but she worked and was on the go a lot. This proved to be a greater challenge than I had anticipated.

About three weeks after my move into the house, an attractive young man came into the alcohol treatment program at the VA where I worked. He was tall, handsome, and slender and had a full head of brownish-auburn hair, complete with sideburns and a mustache, stylish at the time. Kenneth introduced himself in the group therapy session hesitatingly. He often avoided eye contact and failed to participate in discussions. He also attempted to withdraw physically by sitting back away from the inner group circle. The more Kenneth tried to avoid interaction, the more I picked on him in a kidding way. I considered it a personal challenge to draw shy and quiet participants out of their shells and into the group.

We soon learned that Kenneth had a fraternal twin brother and that he was one of nine children, four boys and five girls, who grew up in a small town in south central Virginia. His father worked as a plumber and trained the four boys in the family business. His mother spent most of her time raising the children, cooking, and cleaning. The five girls helped out when they were not in school. It must have been quite a challenge to feed eleven people at one time.

The twin boys, Keith and Kenneth, enlisted in the US Army during the Vietnam War, but both served their active duty in Germany. Keith chose to make a career of the military, but Kenneth served for three years and was then honorably discharged in May of 1966.

Upon returning home from the service, Kenneth began working in the family plumbing business. A year later, he married and soon after started a family. Dwayne was born in August of 1968, and Lisa in August of 1969. Roughly five years later, the marriage ended in divorce and Kenneth's separation from his young children. Kenneth had drinking issues that played a part; however, other significant factors contributed to the breakup. Kenneth spent the next five years searching for answers that would direct him to a better life. This led to his admission into the alcohol treatment program at the Salem VA Hospital.

When he completed the program, Kenneth had no definite plans for the future, but needed a job to get him back on his feet. Like many of the veterans who had no place to go when discharged from the VA, he moved into a nearby halfway house. I would often go over and visit the residents there to see how they were adjusting and progressing with their job searches.

The night Kenneth moved into the halfway house, I was there watching the *Grand Ole Opry* on TV with several of the residents. It was a warm summer evening, and I asked if anyone wanted to go for a milkshake. I had no takers, and returned home without the cherry milkshake I had wanted.

When I called the next day to speak with one of the female veterans I was working with, it just so happened that Kenneth answered the phone. He was the only one there at the time, and to my surprise, he asked if I still wanted that cherry milkshake. Of course, I did. The milkshake and the company were both enjoyable. I found myself attracted to Kenneth, but I'm not sure why. We had little in common. He was shy, and I was outgoing. He was a loner, and I loved having people around. He rarely initiated a conversation, and I could talk to a wall. Maybe opposites do attract.

Kenneth soon got a job, and he and I began spending most evenings and weekends together; eating out or cooking at my place. It made me very happy when Kenneth began going with me to Sunday services and other church activities.

That summer, we attended our annual church picnic which took place at Camp Fincastle. While rowing in a canoe on the lake, I explained to Kenneth the importance of God's presence in my life. I wanted Kenneth to understand that if I had to choose between him and God, God would have to come first. However, I was earnestly praying I would not have to make that decision, since I was growing very fond of Kenneth.

Meanwhile, Kenneth was still struggling with occasional drinking sprees. Following one of these episodes, he called me and said he wanted to give up alcohol. I drove to pick him up, brought him back to my house, and called a male Christian friend to come over for support. As we talked, Kenneth began expressing his feelings of emptiness, loneliness, and insignificance. To him, life seemed hardly worth living. He realized he was at a critical crossroad in his life. He could either head down the same old road or make some major changes. He emptied his beer can down my kitchen sink, and then surrendered his life to Christ. My prayers had been answered!

After that day, Kenneth and I attended church together more regularly. As he became more involved in the various activities, he became more comfortable with himself. Kenneth was well-liked by everyone which helped encourage him in his new walk of faith. A few months later, he officially joined the church. Praise the Lord!

We continued to see each other, and after roughly eight months of dating, we began talking about plans for the future. Following much discussion, we began praying for God to reveal His will for our lives. Prior to this relationship, I had given up on the possibility of marriage; however, I knew that God had placed a lot of love in my heart for some special purpose or person.

MILKSHAKE MADE IN HEAVEN

One warm summer afternoon while on my deck, Kenneth knelt before me and nervously asked, "Now, will you marry me?" I could hardly believe my ears. As I excitedly said, "I will," Kenneth placed a diamond ring on my ring toe. He gently kissed me and assured me he would do all he could to make me happy. I truly thought I could never be any happier than I was at that very moment.

CHAPTER 14

Together in Love

*So they are no longer two, but one.
Therefore what God has joined together,
let man not separate.
Matthew 19:6*

Anxious to share the news, I called my parents and asked them if they could come over for a visit. I'm sure they sensed the excitement in my voice, which raised their curiosity. I told them there was something I wanted them to see. Of course, I was referring to my engagement ring. When Mom and Dad arrived, Kenneth and I shared our good news and explained how we both felt certain that God had brought us together. After our initial discussion, Kenneth took Dad aside to seek his approval. Dad responded, "Just promise me you will be good to her." With that assurance, my parents willingly gave us their blessing.

I had been a participant in many weddings, most often as a soloist and once as the maid of honor, but I had only dreamed of being the bride. Yet another dream was becoming a reality. There was much to do in planning our big day, but as always, my parents were there to help in any way they could.

We chose September 27th of 1980 as our wedding date. It would be my grandmother's eighty-fifth birthday, and we decided it would be appropriate to share our special day with someone who meant so much to both of us. I hated to exclude anyone who wanted to be with us on our wedding day. However, the longer the list grew, the more we realized the need to limit the number of invitations. At the point when I heard that my grandmother's hairdresser wanted to be invited, I realized things had gotten out of control. Limiting the number of invitations naturally simplified the planning process and was a welcome change for my already-shy "husband to be."

Even though our engagement was short, I could hardly wait for the big day to arrive. The wedding took place on a beautiful, clear, fall day. It was mid-afternoon, and the sun shone through the beautiful stained-glass windows of our church. The high-beamed ceiling pointing skyward was a reminder of God's presence with us. The wedding party consisted of six attendants, and a flower girl who were all members of our families. Our faithful minister, Roy Taylor, performed the ceremony. He and his wife, Carol, had become special friends of ours through the years.

My soft-white wedding gown and veil were a gift, specially designed and made by the seamstress who had fitted me so perfectly for years. I wore an orchid corsage, and my Dad escorted me down the aisle and gave me away. Kenneth was quite handsome in his dark blue suit and boutonniere, but his serious and somber expression reflected his nervousness. He was on his knees throughout the ceremony in order for us to be at eye level with each other as we exchanged our vows. He later confessed that he was glad I asked him to kneel, because he felt too wobbly to stand. My matron-of-honor and her husband sang a beautiful song describing a relationship of unending love and commitment. The music added even more warmth and romance to our simple, but meaningful ceremony.

A small reception followed in the fellowship hall where we were showered with gifts and blessings. After cutting and sharing our wedding cake, we all surprised my grandmother by singing "Happy Birthday" while presenting her with a cake of her own. This added a wonderful touch to our special day.

After the reception, Kenneth and I began our honeymoon journey to the Great Smokey Mountains. Cans, streamers, and shaving cream on our van were a sure giveaway that we were newlyweds. We even got a complimentary car wash a few miles down the road.

Our plans were to spend the first night of our honeymoon at the famous Dutch Inn in the small town of Collinsville, Virginia. However, neither of us thought to make reservations due to our preoccupation with the wedding. Upon our arrival, we discovered it was the Martinsville Speedway race weekend, and there was no room in the inn. Not only was the Dutch Inn filled to capacity, but most other motels in the area were also booked. Thankfully, we found an available room a few miles down the road.

The next day, we continued on our journey spending time in historic Winston-Salem and other points of interest along the way. When we reached Gatlinburg and Pigeon Forge, we visited many of the numerous shops and sights. One place we especially enjoyed was Christus Gardens Wax Museum which depicted the story of Jesus' life and ministry while on earth.

The honeymoon was such a special time, and the weather was perfect. The leaves were beginning to turn their beautiful shades. The warm days and cool crisp evenings added to our enjoyment as we began our new life together as husband and wife.

Chapter 15

Married with Children

*Here am I, and the children the
Lord has given me.
Isaiah 8:18a*

Once home from the honeymoon, Kenneth and I began to realize there were more than just a few adjustments to make. My new husband, who was almost six feet tall, had to learn to live in the house built especially for me, with everything at foot level. In addition, we had each grown accustomed to doing things our own way which presented another set of challenges. However, we gradually learned to compromise and make decisions based on what was best for us as a couple.

Less than two years after we were married, just when Kenneth and I had made the necessary adjustments, Kenneth's two children decided they wanted to move in with their dad. Moving two teenagers in with us presented an even greater challenge. I had always wanted to be a mom, but didn't expect it to happen quite this way. Kenneth and I had discussed the idea of having children, prior to getting married. Due to my size, the doctor felt that pregnancy would be difficult, possibly causing me to be bedridden for as much as seven months. This news was more than disappointing; however, considering the doctor's advice, our ages, and the fact that Kenneth already had two children, we decided against having children of our own.

I wasn't quite sure I was prepared for my new role as "stepmom," especially to two teenagers. However, these were Kenneth's children, and because of my love for him, I felt this was the right thing to do. Subsequently, we welcomed these kids into our home and instantly our family of two became a family of four.

At the time the children moved in, Dwayne was close to fifteen years old, and Lisa would soon be fourteen. Both had been living with their mother and stepfather for almost ten years.

Lisa was a sweet and pretty girl with a heart as big as all outdoors. But, it was a difficult time in her life, and she went back and forth deciding whether to live with her mom or her dad. She loved both of her parents, and had idealistic thoughts of getting them back together. This fact made my relationship with Lisa difficult. Whenever I asked her to do anything she didn't want to do, Lisa quickly reminded me that I was not her "real" mom. When her dad was around, however, things were quite different. When I shared this information with Kenneth, he thought I was over-reacting. It didn't help that we often disagreed when it came to disciplinary action.

Whenever there were problems at home or in school, it naturally became my responsibility to deal with them. This caused Lisa to resent me even more, and added to the conflict her dad and I were already experiencing. Things got so bad that Lisa nearly succeeded in coming between her father and me. Kenneth finally had to explain to Lisa that her mom and he would never get back together.

Lisa's brother Dwayne was often my helper in dealing with his sister. Once, for example, Lisa left home because I wouldn't allow her to pierce her own ears without her dad's permission. It was Dwayne who followed after her and persuaded her to return. He stood up for me on many occasions. Just when I was beginning to feel like a stranger in my own home, and tension had about reached the breaking point, Lisa decided to move back in with her mom. I was very disappointed that things had taken this turn, but hoped that this move would lead to a better relationship between Lisa and me.

Dwayne, on the other hand, stayed with us through high school. He was quite handsome and caused us little behavioral problems, but we discovered he was sometimes mischievous and good at covering his tracks. He enjoyed playing pranks on others, especially his dad. Kenneth once found a life-sized witch doll in the kitchen when he came for his morning cup of coffee. On another occasion, wet paper towels were discovered in Kenneth's work boots.

Dwayne and I got along quite well. He was willing to lend a helping hand around the house, and for the most part kept up his grades in school with little effort. He knew how to turn on the charm when it was needed—just like his dad. It seemed only natural for Dwayne to pursue drama in school. He was quite the actor in several of his school plays.

Kenneth and I were very pleased when Dwayne became involved in our youth group at church. These kids became quite close-knit and spent a lot of time together. They studied God's word and attended Christian concerts, retreats and other social events. Dwayne received such great support from this peer group throughout his teenage years.

Chapter 16

Time on the Lake

*The earth is the Lord's, and everything in it, the
world, and all who live in it.*
Psalm 24:1

The year after Lisa moved out, my parents purchased a vacation home on Smith Mountain Lake. This beautiful man-made lake has five hundred miles of shoreline, and is located roughly an hour's drive from home. Mom and Dad's cozy little cottage consisted of a common kitchen and dining area, a living room, three small bedrooms, and one bath. There was an unfinished basement containing a wood stove, hook ups for washer and dryer, and lots of storage space.

I spent most of my time on the full-length deck of the cottage working on my tan. Sometimes, you could find me fishing with a bamboo pole on the dock, occasionally catching a small perch on the line. We all loved our vacation spot, but our view of the lake area from our property was quite limited. This led us to consider buying a boat. After exploring the options, Kenneth and I joined my parents in the purchase of a pontoon boat.

We soon discovered that boating was lots of fun for kids of all ages. My eighty-eight-year-old maternal grandmother amazed us all when she decided to take a ride. The boat provided a great source of entertainment for frequent guests who came to visit with us. Many often brought food to contribute to the delicious meals that Mom, our chief cook, would prepare. There were always those willing to pitch in and help her in the kitchen as needed.

Much of Daddy's time was spent making improvements to the property, and Kenneth often helped. Trees were chopped down, an enclosed porch was added to accommodate more people, and large numbers of rocks were moved and used for landscaping. It always amazed Kenneth how much energy Daddy had for working, often stating that he couldn't keep up with him. Kenneth often jokingly said, "I need to go back to work so that I can get rested up."

Kenneth's plumbing experience came in handy when a basement level bathroom was added to the house. He and Daddy also built a cinderblock chimney to better allow the smoke to escape from the wood stove in the basement. In addition to the changes to the cottage, the existing dock was in such bad condition that they tore it down and replaced it with a larger and much nicer floating dock. Dad also designed a way for them to build a boat ramp and shelter for the pontoon. All these changes added to our special time spent with family and friends at the lake.

Chapter 17

Unexpected Changes

*So do not fear, for I am with you; do not be
dismayed, for I am your God. I will strengthen you
and help you; I will uphold you with
my righteous right hand.*
Isaiah 41:10

Trying to be like everyone else had become a way of life for me. This mindset seemed to be the driving force that kept me going. I was working, driving, married, had children and all was going quite well, until shortly after my fortieth birthday. I'd always heard that "life begins at 40," and I would soon discover what this meant for me.

First of all, both my Aunt Jean and my maternal grandmother had just been diagnosed with cancer. Our family Christmas dinner that year was interrupted by a call from the hospital that my grandmother had taken a turn for the worse from her rare blood cancer. It was spreading rapidly. Most of the family was able to spend a few precious moments with her before she died the morning after Christmas. It was an emotional time for all of us, but we were comforted knowing she was no longer suffering.

The day after my grandmother's funeral, I was doing my usual household chores, specifically using a Bissell carpet sweeper. My left leg became extremely tired and ached with pain. I just thought the stressors of the past few weeks and days were catching up with me. But the next morning I could neither bend nor straighten my leg, and the pain in my knee was increasing. Realizing I must have over done it, I decided to rest and give it a few days to heal.

When things didn't improve, I scheduled an appointment with my faithful orthopedic physician. Dr. Bray reminded me that what most people ordinarily do using two arms and two legs, I had accomplished by using only my one leg. My left knee had degenerated from overuse, and there was a strong possibility I would no longer be able to hyperextend it to perform my daily tasks. For many years, working and striving for independence had been a way of life for me. Unfortunately, I never stopped to consider the consequences of pushing myself to be like everyone else. Dr. Bray was very familiar with how I had made adjustments in learning to compensate for my physical limitations throughout the years. At his recommendation, an appointment was made for me to be evaluated at the UVA Hospital in Charlottesville, Virginia.

The news concerning my knee was devastating. My physical pain was suddenly overshadowed by an overwhelming emotional response. I, like most people, had taken for granted many things in my life. I had been doing most of my own bathing, dressing, and personal grooming. Now, I couldn't even feed myself. What would I do now? I gradually began to feel a sense of helplessness and hopelessness.

For the first time in my life, I considered myself handicapped. I became quite angry and despondent, even questioning God. "Why me Lord and why now?" I had always worked hard at being "normal," and took pride in my accomplishments. How would I suddenly go from striving to be independent to learning to be dependent on others? It wouldn't be easy, but I knew in my heart that I still had a choice. I could choose to be defeated and give up, or I could accept this major setback as yet another challenge and move forward. I chose the latter, but realized I couldn't do it alone. I needed help; physical, emotional, and spiritual. Most of all, I needed God's loving hands to encourage and guide me.

At my initial appointment in Charlottesville, Dr. Whitehill felt I could benefit from in-patient therapy at their Towers Rehab Unit.

I was a little apprehensive, especially at the thought of being away from Kenneth for the first time since we were married. However, at the prospect of regaining some of my independence, I decided to participate in the program.

When Kenneth left me the day I entered the Towers Rehab Center, I thought my heart was breaking. While peering out of a window, tears were streaming down my cheeks as Kenneth waved goodbye, and drove away. I knew, however, that God had given me this opportunity, and I was determined to do my best so that Kenneth's and my separation would be as brief as possible. It didn't take me long to get acquainted with patients and staff, and join in the program. I was now driven by the new challenges I faced.

Through intense physical and occupational therapy, I learned new ways of taking care of myself, regaining much of my strength and functioning ability. Once again, I could bathe myself, comb my hair, brush my teeth, and even do some of my own dressing with the aid of adaptive sticks and gadgets.

After twelve days of therapy, I was extremely happy to see Kenneth and return home to practice all the things I had learned. One thing I never quite mastered was being able to feed myself. I tried really hard to use the long-handled fork and spoon they adapted for me. But without my previous dexterity and coordination, it became too frustrating for me to balance and maneuver the food on the utensil into my mouth. Although I was determined to feed myself, more often than not, the food landed on the table or floor. Adjusting to the need for others to feed me would by far be the most difficult change for me to accept.

Chapter 18

Major Adjustments

*Trust in the Lord with all your heart and lean not
on your own understanding; in all your
ways acknowledge him, and he will
make your paths straight.*
Proverbs 3:5-6

I had accumulated a sizable amount of leave from my job at the VA which enabled me time to consider how my physical changes would affect my work. Meanwhile, I decided to apply for employee disability benefits despite being told how difficult it was to obtain. This involved roughly six months of tedious paperwork and doctors' recommendations.

Sandwiched between my last day at work and my official retirement, Kenneth and I had the wonderful opportunity to travel to Hawaii with our neighbors Dickie and Gail. This was the perfect pick-me-up following my injury. Although the flights were long and tiring, we were soon filled with a renewed sense of energy as we landed on the island. Each passenger was greeted with a beautiful and fragrant lei of flowers. This traditional warm greeting heightened our excitement as we began our vacation.

Our emotions quickly changed when we discovered that my custom made wheelchair which had been checked with our luggage failed to arrive at our destination. The airline compensated us with the use of a standard size chair which clearly didn't fit my needs. At my tallest and with a little stretch of the imagination, I might measure four feet and four inches in height. My feet dangled several inches from the ground, preventing me from maneuvering myself around as I normally would. In this situation, I was forced to rely on someone else to get me where I needed to go. Fortunately, my chair was delivered to the hotel the following day which greatly improved my spirits. With a good night's rest and the arrival of my own *handy* chair, we were excited and anxious to *really* begin our adventure in Hawaii.

One vivid memory for Gail and me occurred as we sat in the sand on Waikiki Beach. While peacefully enjoying the sights, sounds and smells of the Island, a large wave suddenly engulfed us. Evidently, the surf was coming in and we were in the ideal spot to be manipulated by nature's high tide. We laughed hysterically as the water splashed against us filling our mouths with saltiness as we continued to be tossed by the waves. Once the waves rolled back into the sea, our swimsuits were filled with large amounts of sand. Later, Kenneth and I had another good laugh as the sand from the swimsuit filled the bathtub while washing up from our time on the beach.

Our plans also took us to the very tropical island of Kauai. While there, we scheduled a helicopter tour of the island. The anticipation of this adventure created a mixture of emotions, both excitement and nervousness. However, this breathtaking experience became the highlight of our entire week. The views of the beautiful canyons and waterfalls were indescribable.

Soon after returning home from our paradise vacation, I was pleasantly surprised to learn that my disability application had been approved. Suddenly, I was faced with many thoughts concerning what to do now that I would no longer be working.

Then came my official retirement from the VA Medical Center. The EEO (Equal Employment Opportunity) held a luncheon for me at the beautiful La Maison restaurant in Roanoke. On another occasion, Kathy, a coworker and friend who had also graduated in my class at Emory and Henry, held a farewell reception in my honor at the VA. It was a heartwarming send-off; and I was amazed that so many friends, family, and coworkers came to celebrate my fourteen years of civil service.

After my retirement in 1985, life changed for Kenneth and for me. Because of my new limitations, he had taken on many additional responsibilities in the home, and felt more and more tied down. At the same time, I was searching for a new identity and purpose. This resulted in stress for each of us, and consequently put strain on our relationship. Roanoke experienced a devastating flood at this time which seemed highly symbolic of the losses and overflow of emotions Kenneth and I were both experiencing. As a result of the sudden onset of this flood, it took Kenneth four hours to return home from a routine trip to the nearby grocery store.

Being home and alone was not a good match for my personality. Anticipating the need for activity and being with others, I had already arranged to volunteer with Easter Seals once a week. I served in the Parent Infant Education Program (PIEP) as a facilitator for a group of parents with physically challenged infants and toddlers. My job was to initiate conversation so that those attending could encourage, and support each other. I enjoyed this, but it didn't seem to satisfy my personal longing for something more. After volunteering for nearly two years, I decided to try something else.

Around this same time period, many family things were happening. Dwayne graduated from high school and many of his friends were going to college. Although Dwayne was somewhat influenced by their decisions, he stuck with his original plan and enlisted in the US Army. Soon after his eighteenth birthday, Kenneth drove Dwayne to the bus station where he would leave for his military training at Fort McClellan, Alabama. Lisa married and had our first grandchild, Jessica, who was born in March of 1987. Kenneth and I adjusted quite well as grandparents and welcomed this new and positive role in our lives.

With no children living in the house, the conflict in our marriage was much harder to avoid. Kenneth occasionally turned to drinking as an escape which led to more insecurity in our relationship. Clearly, my ability to serve as wife and homemaker had drastically changed causing me to wonder if my added limitations were contributing to Kenneth's desire to drink.

Kenneth's drinking most often took place during his occasional fishing trips with his brother. But, the anticipation of facing the next episode was always in the back of my mind. Even worse than the *episode* was the emotional distance that drinking put between us. Kenneth was aware of my disapproval which in turn made me feel alienated from the most important person in my life. He continued taking care of me, and fulfilling his responsibilities in our home; however, there was an obvious distance in our relationship.

Recognizing my need for healthy adult interaction, I took the suggestion from one of the PIEP leaders at Easter Seals to attend a women's Bible study called Bible Study Fellowship. BSF is an international and interdenominational study of God's Word. Feeling loved and accepted by this group of ladies greatly improved my outlook, and gave me new hope. Although I had read the Bible and attended church all my life, this study sparked a significant desire for more insight into God's Word. I felt more like myself again, and my relationship with God became more alive and personal in a way I had never experienced.

More family changes occurred with Dwayne's marriage, and the birth of his first child. Jesse was born in August of 1989 while his father was still serving in Germany as a military policeman. After being discharged from the Army, his family came to live with Kenneth and me for about a month while searching for a house of their own. Shortly after settling into their new home, Dwayne landed a position with the Police Department in our area. Kenneth and I were happy to have Dwayne and his family nearby.

For a short period of time, I volunteered as a group facilitator back at the VA. I enjoyed the time spent with old coworkers, but upon hearing about an opportunity to work with physically and mentally challenged children in a local elementary school, I decided to offer my time there. I worked once a week as a teacher's assistant, and enjoyed interacting with the children. Because this position required a lot of hands-on instruction, my personal involvement was somewhat limited. After volunteering a year and a half, I decided to leave this position so that I could spend more time with family.

Chapter 19

Searching for Purpose

*For I know the plans I have for you, declares the
Lord, plans to prosper you and not to harm you,
plans to give you hope and a future.*
Jeremiah 29:11

In October of 1990, my friend Kathy and I were privileged to attend a retreat held in Pennsylvania and hosted by Joni Eareckson. Joni is well-known for her amazing accomplishments despite paralysis brought on by a diving accident she experienced as a young teenager. Her story had become a great inspiration to me. In fact, I had corresponded with Joni prior to knowing of this event hoping that we might someday meet face-to-face.

When Kathy and I entered the large fully packed room at the retreat, she insisted that we sit up front allowing for the best view. As Joni entered the stage, she spotted me in the crowd. When our eyes met and she mouthed, "Hello Norma," I was thrilled beyond words. To my surprise, Joni had prearranged a private meeting for us following the event so that we could become more acquainted. This special time spent with her greatly inspired me to use my life in a way that is encouraging to others, especially those feeling hopeless.

Kenneth and I had purchased a Subaru not long before the retreat. Kathy and I were hoping to take it on our trip, but Kenneth was concerned that something might happen to his car with the two of us in charge. So we traveled in Kathy's vehicle instead. Our trip up went rather smoothly. However, while traveling home, somehow we got turned around in the wrong direction and wound up going around the I-495 Beltway of Washington DC during rush hour traffic. We got very tickled over our unfortunate mistake, but refused to let it dampen our fun time. When we finally arrived home, and pulled into my driveway, Kathy and I noticed that the Subaru windshield was covered with cardboard. Kenneth met us outside and explained that while traveling to his mother's, a turkey had flown through the windshield, shattering it into pieces. Kathy and I laughed and said, "And you didn't want *us* to take your car, because *we* might damage it?" We've had a lot of fun with this story.

The following year, July 1991, Kenneth and I attended another one of Joni Eareckson's retreats. This Spruce Lake Retreat was held in the Pocono Mountains of Pennsylvania. We met many wonderful people during our time there, including Joni's husband Ken Tada. The retreat functioned as a support group for families with children or spouses having special needs. Help, encouragement, and support were extended to the caregivers as well as those receiving care. Having this experience gave Kenneth and me a refreshing and new perspective in our own situation.

It was also during this summer we celebrated my Dad's seventy-fifth birthday, with many friends and family. Unfortunately, Dad began experiencing health issues a few months later which required a heart catheterization followed by angioplasty. We were very pleased that he did well through these procedures and quickly resumed his normal and active lifestyle.

Around this time, one of the couples we met in the Poconos mailed us a photograph from their hometown newspaper concerning a young boy named Jacob with physical features very similar to my own. Although the article contained very little information, I was super excited to know about this child and his family and was determined to locate them. Persistence paid off when I finally spoke with Jacob's mother on the phone. She was elated to talk with someone who was so much like her son, and was quite interested in knowing how I had adapted and coped with the unique challenges in my life. I was just as excited to hear about Jacob and more than willing to share any helpful information. Not long after our phone conversation, we were privileged to meet face-to-face in each other's homes.

Still searching for productive ways to spend my time, I pursued hobbies and activities I never seemed to have time to do while working full-time. In addition to spending time with my grandchildren, I enjoyed taking voice lessons, occasionally singing for friends' weddings, community events and church services. I also began cross-stitching, amazing many with my "foot-craftsmanship" as well as my ability to thread a needle. Cross-stitching was a great stay-at-home activity, but I missed getting out and spending time with others. I had completed the five studies offered by BSF, and stopped attending so that others on a waiting list could participate. However, I missed the structured study of God's word and the fellowship it provided.

A welcomed event occurred with the birth of Dwayne's second child, Brittany, in December of 1992. Kenneth and I were proud and happy to welcome another grandchild into our lives. This gave me more opportunity to interact with family; however, I still felt a yearning for something else in my life.

Chapter 20

Trying Times

And we know that in all things God works for the good of those who love him, who have been called according to his purpose.
Romans 8:28

In the spring of 1993, I crossed paths with someone I had known in church many years ago. She and I began to spend time together discovering that we enjoyed doing a lot of the same things. We quickly became close friends, talking at length on the phone and going many places together. This relationship enabled me to do a lot of the things that I had not done for a long period of time, which certainly helped lift my spirits.

Meanwhile, Lisa had her second child, Jeffrey, in December of 1993. Although Kenneth and I were once again happy to be grandparents, things between the two of us were not improving. Many times since my retirement, I had suggested to him that we go for counseling, but Kenneth always responded with, "I thought we were doing ok." His response only discouraged me more by proving how differently we viewed the situation. As if our relationship was not strained enough, I began experiencing the onset of menopause and many heightened emotions.

Seeing no positive changes in our marriage, I decided to seek counseling on my own. After several sessions, it became clear that my relationship with my new best friend was affecting my interaction with my husband and my family even more than I realized. My needs were being satisfied within my friendship while Kenneth's needs were inadvertently being placed on the sidelines. I realized then that I needed to make a healthy change for the sake of my marriage.

Subsequently, my friend and I began spending less time together, and I decided to get back into BSF. While reconnecting socially with the ladies in bible study, I realized how much healthier these relationships were for me and for my marriage. Over the next few years, I gradually regained my positive outlook and lifestyle. This involved working through feelings of guilt and regret over past mistakes and grasping the truth of what was most important in my life. Despite personal progress, things between Kenneth and I had unfortunately not shown many signs of improvement.

CHAPTER 21

Hope

*The Lord is good to those whose hope is in him,
to the one who seeks him.*
Lamentations 3:25

In September of 1995, Kenneth went to Edisto Beach in South Carolina to fish with his brother. Within that same timeframe, a couple of my friends and I decided we would take a girls' trip to Virginia Beach. This impromptu decision helped ease my concerns over Kenneth's trip, and the drinking that might take place.

From beginning to end, the girls' beach escape was both relaxing and filled with laughter. When we returned home, I was surprised to see Kenneth there earlier than expected. He later explained that during his trip, the whole drinking scene had lost its appeal. I was encouraged by this news which gave me renewed hope for our marriage.

The following year, Kenneth's summer trip to fish with Roger felt different to him. He began his time there drinking his usual beer, but a few days into the trip he switched to Dr. Pepper. Kenneth felt there had to be more to life than what he was experiencing. Ironically, the last night spent at Roger's, they watched a TV program depicting the biblical character Moses. Before going to sleep that evening, many thoughts rushed through his mind, including how his drinking had played a significant role in the unhealthy condition of our relationship. Kenneth faced yet another major crossroad in his life. Fortunately, he made the decision to give up alcohol and focus on our marriage.

In 1997, Kenneth had planned another vacation to fish with Roger. Meanwhile, several of my BSF girlfriends and I were planning to attend a Christian women's conference on the same weekend. These ladies were somewhat aware of the troubles in my marriage, and consequently prayed with me that God would intervene and Kenneth's plans would change. Upon returning from the conference, we asked Kenneth about his fishing trip. It was then that we discovered he had not taken the trip because of an unexpected stomach issue. Obviously, this was not the response we had anticipated or even hoped for, but we knew God had answered our prayers. This personal experience with God added a special ending to our uplifting weekend.

During the months that followed, a friend from church had been encouraging Kenneth to join him in the men's group of BSF. This came at a time when Kenneth was earnestly seeking answers. After giving this long and serious consideration, he decided to give it a try at the beginning of the New Year. As mentioned earlier, the men's and women's groups cover the same material, enabling Kenneth and me to share and discuss what we were learning each week. I was excited and optimistic about the effect this might have on our relationship.

Chapter 22

Seniors on the Go

*The Lord has done great things for us,
and we are filled with joy.*
Psalm 126:3

It was becoming increasingly more difficult for me to manage things alone at home. One particular day while Kenneth was at work, I was transferring into my wheelchair and missed the seat. Instead, I landed onto the footrest, and after several unsuccessful attempts to lift myself up, I slid to the floor. I scooted down the long hallway from the bathroom to the kitchen phone. Catching my breath, I lifted the receiver to the floor, placed my ear against it and used my toes to dial my neighbor. This was done by touch since I couldn't visibly see the top of the phone. Thankfully, my neighbor was home and willing to come to my rescue. Huffing, puffing, and waddling to the back door, I reached up to unlock it by lying on my back. After all this, I was shocked when she unexpectedly knocked on my *front* door. Dampened with sweat and using my last bit of energy, I managed to reach the other door and unlock it. When she opened it and looked down at me, she asked, "What are you doing down there?" She and I immediately burst into uncontrollable laughter.

After this and other similar instances, Kenneth and I began discussing the need for additional help at home. Some of the options we considered were adult day care, hiring outside help, or requesting assistance from family and friends. After looking at these more closely, we came up with yet another option. Kenneth decided that taking early retirement would be the best possible solution. This was a win-win decision since he was more than willing to retire, and I would certainly benefit from having him at home.

Once Kenneth was retired, we began spending more time with our now five grandchildren who frequently stayed overnight with us. Dwayne's third child, Lance, was two years old at this time. We also traveled more, often taking my parents along. I continued singing in our church choir, and we both served as church Elders. Kenneth and I participated in the seniors group appropriately called "Seniors on the Go." We both attended the church prayer meetings weekly, and I became involved in an organization called Rafiki Foundation supporting orphan children in Africa. We both continued in Bible Study Fellowship, and our friends there convinced us to join yet another seniors' group called "Golden Friends."

These were good active years during which Kenneth and I slowly, but surely were making progress towards a healthier marriage. We welcomed this season of our lives and the new special friendships we developed.

Chapter 23

Reversal of Roles

*Children's children are a crown to the aged, and
parents are the pride of their children.*
Proverbs 17:6

Mom and Dad lived near us, and it was not unusual for them to stop by for a visit when they were out and about, often bringing things from the store that we needed. However, as their health began declining this happened less frequently. They themselves began to recognize their increasing limitations and need for assistance. As a result, Mom and Dad began discussing other possible living options.

Meanwhile, Mom held an open house celebration for Dad in honor of his ninetieth birthday. Many family and friends came to share this milestone with him. Not long after this joyous occasion, Mom and Dad shared with us their plans to move into an assisted living facility. Their house went on the market and sold surprisingly fast. Within two and a half months, they were in their new home. Unfortunately, two days later, Dad was taken to the hospital emergency room due to the stress brought on by this sudden major change. He was given something to settle his nerves and sent home to rest. Dad knew he and mom had made the right decision to move, but had not expected things to happen so quickly.

REVERSAL OF ROLES

Less than a month later, my mother-in-law passed away at the age of ninety-two. Kenneth had a sweet and caring relationship with his mother. They often said things to make each other laugh. During the end of one of our visits, Kenneth mentioned that we needed to get on the road before dark. Mom responded, "What's the matter? Doesn't your car have lights?" We would truly miss our monthly trips to Charlotte County to spend time with her. We began these visits even before we were married. I am thankful to have known both of Kenneth's parents before their departure from this world, sharing four years with his father before his passing in 1983 and many more years with his mom. After losing both of his parents, Kenneth adopted my parents as his own. In many ways he already felt much like a son to them.

Two months after my parents settled into their new home, Mom suffered a broken right leg and hip due to an accidental fall. This required surgery and several weeks of therapy in another nursing home. Daddy struggled with being separated from his sweetheart, and managed to be there with her for much of the time. They had a very special kind of love. He was by far the happiest upon her return to their new three room apartment at the retirement home.

Roughly a year later, Dad stopped driving; therefore, Kenneth and Barry began providing transportation to and from their appointments. In addition, Dad began experiencing bouts of pneumonia and required oxygen on a regular basis, although not always following the doctor's orders. I caught him on several occasions not hooked up, and on other occasions with tubes haphazardly in place. He had a special way of responding when I brought this to his attention, shooting one of his sheepish grins my way.

Four years later, Mom experienced another broken hip that required skilled care not available at her and Dad's residence. Therefore, she was transferred into a rehab center for therapy. We soon learned progressive care was available there, meaning all levels of care could be accommodated. Because of this, we all decided it would be best to move Dad there too. This became their new home, and enabled them to be in the same facility no matter what level of care they needed.

This proved to be a good decision. Within six weeks of Dad's move, he fell and broke *his* hip. Over the next eight months, Dad was in and out of the hospital and rehab on three different occasions. He and Mom were finally able to live together in their apartment for roughly five and a half months. Dad then returned to the hospital with pneumonia. Soon after being released and returned to rehab, my dear daddy left this world on April 5, 2013. Evidently, his heart just gave out at the age of ninety-five.

My parents came *so* close to celebrating their seventy-fifth year of marriage. What an inspirational example their love was to so many people. They were selected to be crowned King and Queen of Hearts at their nursing home residence on their last Valentine's Day together. What an appropriate recognition for these two special people in my life.

CHAPTER 24

God's Hands, Not Mine

*I remember the days of long ago; I meditate
on all your works and consider
what your hands have done.
Psalm 143:5*

Looking back, I can see the many ways God's hands have provided for me. Even before my birth, God had specifically chosen the parents best suited for my needs. This has been a significant factor in my life. In the beginning, Mom and Dad wholeheartedly sought God's guidance for the strength, encouragement, and wisdom they needed. If my parents had taken the doctor's advice; things could have been quite different for me.. In Philippians 4:5b-7 the Bible states, *The Lord is near. Do not be anxious about anything, but in every situation, by prayers and petition, with thanksgiving, present your requests to God. And the peace of God, which transcends all understanding, will guard your hearts and your minds in Christ Jesus.*

Our home was built on biblical principles and God's love. As a result, my parents dedicated me to the Lord when I was almost two years old, promising with the help of the people in our church to raise me in a Christian environment.

My maternal grandparents were also very active in our church. Granddaddy Pritchett regularly studied God's word, taught Sunday school, and served in leadership for many years. I looked up to him and Grandma, learning a lot about Christian living by their example.

My fraternal grandparents were also members of our church prior to their move to Portsmouth, Virginia. I have no memory of my Granddaddy Milam since I was only two when he passed away. However, I am often reminded of him by the handicap ramp he built to assist the aging members of our church. At that time, he had no idea that this ramp would one day be used by his own granddaughter. God clearly provided for me in this way as well.

In addition to my family's influence, I learned a lot about the Bible in Sunday school and church. As a result of my knowing God and His love for me, I made the personal decision to accept Jesus Christ as my Lord and Savior. I was only eleven years old when I proclaimed my faith and had no idea what a huge difference this would make regarding my future.

As a youth through Christian Endeavor, I learned much more about God's word and how to apply it. Incidentally, this was the same Christian group in which as teenagers my parents were introduced to one another some thirty years earlier. At the age of fifteen, Dad was invited to attend Mom's church one evening, and in his words, saw "the prettiest little girl he had ever seen." Six years later, he asked for her hand in marriage. It is clear to me that God was at work, even then.

Not only did God bless me with great Christian influences, but He also gave me an optimistic and outgoing personality which positively affected how I perceived and reacted to the challenges I faced. My sense of humor was especially helpful in awkward or uncomfortable situations. And because I was persistent, or should I say stubborn, nothing seemed to prevent me from doing the things I really wanted to do.

From my experiences at Camp Easter Seal, I learned to set goals based on my own expectations, rather than on what everyone else was doing. This was a huge stepping stone for me, which gave me the freedom to be more like the person God created me to be. This new insight and the special friendships I formed at camp gave me the encouragement and confidence I needed to pursue a college education.

After graduating from Emory and Henry, it amazed me how quickly God directed me to a job I would never have pursued on my own. Working at the VA was a good fit for me, and provided benefits far beyond my expectations. I got the job in 1971, my van in 1974, my house in 1979, my husband in 1980, and children in 1982. Only God could have orchestrated such a plan. Ephesians 3:20 states, *Now to Him who is able to do immeasurably more than all we ask or imagine, according to His power that is at work within us.*

Things seemed to be going so well, until my knee injury. Suddenly, everything changed and I began questioning God. Why was He allowing this to happen? I struggled through this time, but never turned my back on God. It was difficult to let go of the independent mindset that for so long had motivated my actions. However, as I wrestled with God, He gradually revealed to me that nothing I had accomplished in the past had happened without His intervention.

God was the one who had provided earthly hands to come to my aid when I needed them. While searching for new identity and purpose, God encouraged me to simply live out the things I had been taught from His word. He was with me before the injury, and He would be with me now. His ultimate desire was for me to be fully dependent on Him. When I accepted this, I began to experience the peace and contentment that comes from doing the will of God. Philippians 4:9 tells us, *Whatever you have learned or received or heard from me or seen in me—put it into practice. And the God of peace will be with you.*

It is clear to me now that Kenneth's involvement in BSF marked the beginning of small and gradual improvements in *our* relationship. Through Bible study, Kenneth and I gained a better knowledge and understanding of God's presence in our lives. It was God working in each of us that brought us to a stronger and healthier place in our marriage. *And we know that in all things God works for the good of those who love Him, which have been called according to His purpose* (Romans 8:28).

Kenneth and I were surprised and honored to receive the "King and Queen of Hearts" award at our church's 2015 Sweetheart Dinner. This meant so much to me as I recalled the 2013 Valentine's Day celebration at Mom and Dad's nursing home.

My relationship with Dwayne and Lisa has also been greatly enriched through the years. Despite my and Lisa's beginning, we now share a very special mother-daughter bond. I thank God for the blessing of these children.

There are many verses from God's word that have had an impact on my life; however, the one that has given me the most encouragement and comfort is found in Psalm 139:13-14. It says, *For you created my inmost being; you knit me together in my mother's womb. I praise you because I am fearfully and wonderfully made; your works are wonderful, I know that full well.* Appropriately so, I introduced these words to you at the beginning of my life story.

Now, when I consider the two verses that follow, I see how appropriate they are for the ending. Psalm 139:15–16 states, *My frame was not hidden from you when I was made in the secret place. When I was woven together in the depths of the earth, your eyes saw my unformed body. All the days ordained for me were written in your book before one of them came to be.* God knew everything about me before I was born and had a plan for my life even then. How amazing is God!

Despite God's activity in my life, I can still struggle at times with concerns about who will care for me if something happens to Kenneth. During these times, I am quick to remind myself of how faithful God has been throughout my journey in this world. He comforts me with the words in Deuteronomy 31:8 which say, *The Lord Himself goes before you and will go with you; He will never leave you nor forsake you. Do not be afraid; do not be discouraged.*

I choose to believe this in addition to God's promise in Philippians 1:6 which states, *Being confident of this, that He who began a good work in you will carry it on to completion until the day of Christ Jesus.* This truth gives me the assurance that God will care for me until the day I see Him face to face.

God is so good! He has led me through this entire process of sharing my story with you. I pray that you know God. His love for you is greater than you could ever imagine, and His greatest desire is that *you* have a close relationship with Him through His Son, Jesus Christ. All you need to do is believe; believe that God sent Jesus into the world to provide a way for us to be with Him always. *If you confess with your mouth, "Jesus is Lord," and believe in your heart that God raised Him from the dead, you will be saved* (Romans 10:9).

GOD'S HANDS NOT MINE

As he went along,
he saw a man blind from birth.
His disciples asked him, 'Rabbi, who sinned,
This man or his parents, that he was born blind?
Neither this man nor his parents sinned,' said Jesus,
'but this happened so that the works of God
might be displayed in him.
John 9:1–3

God's Hands, Not Mine

Written by Kathryn Cole

Verse 1
All my life I've been God's child, dependent on His grace.
In everyone who lends a hand, I see my Father's face.
My hopes and dreams, my plans and goals,
were nurtured by His Word
That those in faith could trust in Him and
know their prayers were heard.

Chorus
My life is in God's hands, I know.
He carries me wherever I go.
When life seems hard to bear, I feel His touch divine.
For my life is in God's hands, not mine.

Verse 2
I never could have done alone, what God would have me do.
He helps me carry out my plans through deeds of friends like you.
Whenever there were hills to climb or views I could not see,
God worked through earthly angels who
stretched out their hands to me.

(Chorus)

Verse 3
I praise His name for leading me to live abundantly,
For giving me a voice to sing and eyes to clearly see.
My greatest joy and gratitude comes when I find it's true
That God is lending you a hand when I reach out to you.

(Chorus)

The music and lyrics to this song were written in the mid '90s by my college and VA friend Kathy. I had the pleasure of singing and sharing it on several occasions.

ABOUT THE AUTHOR

Writing a book had never entered the mind of Norma Garrett, until her dad, one day, made the suggestion. Although she was born without arms and several other disabilities, Norma oddly never considered herself "handicapped" until an injury changed everything. It was at this point that she discovered a much deeper relationship with God. As a result, Norma was given the strength and courage to accept the changes in her life knowing full well that God would always be with her.

CPSIA information can be obtained
at www.ICGtesting.com
Printed in the USA
FSOW01n1613301117
41558FS